Complete Keto Air Fryer Cooking Guide

Super Simple and Delicious Meat Recipes for Beginners

Rudy Kent

© **Copyright 2020 - All rights reserved.**

The content contained within this book may not be reproduced, duplicated or transmitted without direct written permission from the author or the publisher.

Under no circumstances will any blame or legal responsibility be held against the publisher, or author, for any damages, reparation, or monetary loss due to the information contained within this book. Either directly or indirectly.

Legal Notice:

This book is copyright protected. This book is only for personal use. You cannot amend, distribute, sell, use, quote or paraphrase any part, or the content within this book, without the consent of the author or publisher.

Disclaimer Notice:

Please note the information contained within this document is for educational and entertainment purposes only. All effort has been executed to present accurate, up to date, and reliable, complete information. No warranties of any kind are declared or implied. Readers acknowledge that the author is not engaging in the rendering of legal, financial, medical or professional advice. The content within this book has been derived from various sources. Please consult a licensed professional before attempting any techniques outlined in this book.

By reading this document, the reader agrees that under no circumstances is the author responsible for any losses, direct or indirect, which are incurred as a result of the use of information contained within this document, including, but not limited to, — errors, omissions, or inaccuracies.

Introduction

What's the difference between an air fryer and deep fryer? Air fryers bake food at a high temperature with a high-powered fan, while deep fryers cook food in a vat of oil that has been heated up to a specific temperature. Both cook food quickly, but an air fryer requires practically zero preheat time while a deep fryer can take upwards of 10 minutes. Air fryers also require little to no oil and deep fryers require a lot that absorb into the food. Food comes out crispy and juicy in both appliances, but don't taste the same, usually because deep fried foods are coated in batter that cook differently in an air fryer vs a deep fryer. Battered foods needs to be sprayed with oil before cooking in an air fryer to help them color and get crispy, while the hot oil soaks into the batter in a deep fryer. Flour-based batters and wet batters don't cook well in an air fryer, but they come out very well in a deep fryer.

The ketogenic diet is one such example. The diet calls for a very small number of carbs to be eaten. This means food such as rice, pasta, and other starchy vegetables like potatoes are off the menu. Even relaxed versions of the keto diet minimize carbs to a large extent and this compromises the goals of many dieters. They end up having to exert large amounts of willpower to follow the diet. This doesn't do them any favors since willpower is like a muscle. At some point, it tires and this is when the dieter goes right back to their old pattern of eating. I have personal experience with this. In terms of health benefits, the keto diet offers the most. The reduction of carbs forces your body to mobilize fat and this results in automatic fat loss and better health.

Feel free to mix and match the recipes you see in here and play around with them. Eating is supposed to be fun! Unfortunately, we've associated fun eating with unhealthy food. This doesn't have to be the case. The air fryer, combined with the Mediterranean diet, will make your mealtimes fun-filled again and full of taste. There's no grease and messy cleanups to deal with anymore. Are you excited yet?

You should be! You're about to embark on a journey full of air fried goodness!

Table of Contents

Introduction 5

Gruyère Chicken with Lemon 9
Apricot & Garlic Chicken Breasts 10
Restaurant-Style Chicken with Yogurt 13
One-Tray Parmesan Chicken Wings 15
Crunchy Coconut Chicken Dippers 17
Chicken Fillets with Sweet Chili Adobo 19
Avocado & Mango Chicken Breasts 21
Ham & Cheese Filled Chicken Breasts 23
Tasty Chicken Kiev 25
Sweet Mustard Chicken Thighs 27
Thyme-Fried Chicken Legs 29
Honey-Glazed Turkey 30
Spice-Rubbed Jerk Chicken Wings 33
Sweet Sesame Chicken Wings 35
Crispy Breaded Chicken Breasts 37
Crispy Chicken Tenderloins 39
Gluten-Free Crunchy Chicken 41
Gingery Chicken Wings 43
Rosemary & Oyster Chicken Breasts 45
Chicken Thighs with Parmesan Crust 47
Chicken & Baby Potato Traybake 49
Portuguese Roasted Whole Chicken 51
Turkey & Veggie Skewers 53
Chipotle Buttered Turkey 55
Sweet Curried Chicken Cutlets 57

Chicken Thighs with Herby Tomatoes 59

BBQ Whole Chicken... 61

Thyme Turkey Nuggets.. 63

Hot Chili Chicken Wings... 65

Homemade Chicken Patties.. 67

Chicken Pinchos with Salsa Verde 69

Juicy Chicken Fillets with Peppers 71

Crumbed Sage Chicken Scallopini.. 73

Hawaiian-Style Chicken 75

Garlicky Chicken on Green Bed 77

Hot Green Curry Chicken Drumsticks 79

Whole Chicken with Sage & Garlic... 81

Parmesan Turkey Meatballs 83

Turkey Stuffed Bell Peppers 85

Authentic Mongolian Chicken Wings... 87

Spiced Chicken Tacos... 89

Harissa Chicken Sticks... 91

Chicken Breasts en Papillote... 93

Paprika Chicken Breasts.. 95

Caprese Chicken with Balsamic Sauce 97

Buttermilk Chicken Thighs.. 99

Sweet & Sticky Chicken Drumsticks... 101

Turkey Fingers with Cranberry Glaze.. 103

Chicken Skewers with Yogurt Dip 105

Popcorn Chicken Tenders.. 107

Gruyère Chicken with Lemon

Cooking Time:
20 minutes

Serve: 4

Ingredients:
½ cup seasoned breadcrumbs
¼ cup Gruyere cheese, grated
1 lb chicken breasts
½ cup flour
2 eggs, beaten
Salt and black pepper to taste
4 lemon slices

Directions:
1. Preheat air fryer to 370 F. Spray the air fryer basket with cooking spray.

2. Mix the breadcrumbs with Gruyere cheese in a bowl, beat the eggs in another bowl, and add the flour to a third bowl.

3. Toss the chicken in the flour, then in the eggs, and then in the breadcrumb mixture. Place in the frying basket and Air Fry for 12-14 minutes. At the 6-minute mark, turn the chicken over.

4. Once golden brown, remove to a plate and serve topped with lemon slices.

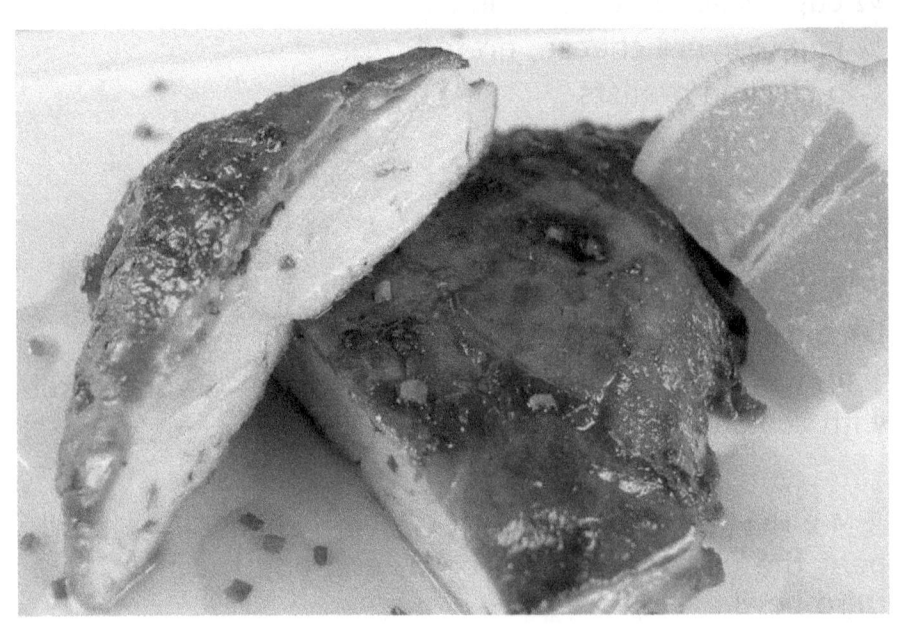

Apricot & Garlic Chicken Breasts

Cooking Time:

22 minutes

Serve: 4

Ingredients:

1 tsp yellow mustard
1 tbsp apricot jam
2 garlic cloves, minced
Salt and black pepper to taste
1 lb chicken breasts
3 tbsp butter, melted

Directions:

1. Preheat air fryer to 360 F. In a bowl, combine together mustard, butter, garlic, apricot jam, black pepper, and salt; mix well.

2. Rub the chicken with the mixture and place it in the greased air fryer basket. Bake for 10 minutes, flip,

and cook for 5-6 more minutes until crispy. Slice before serving.

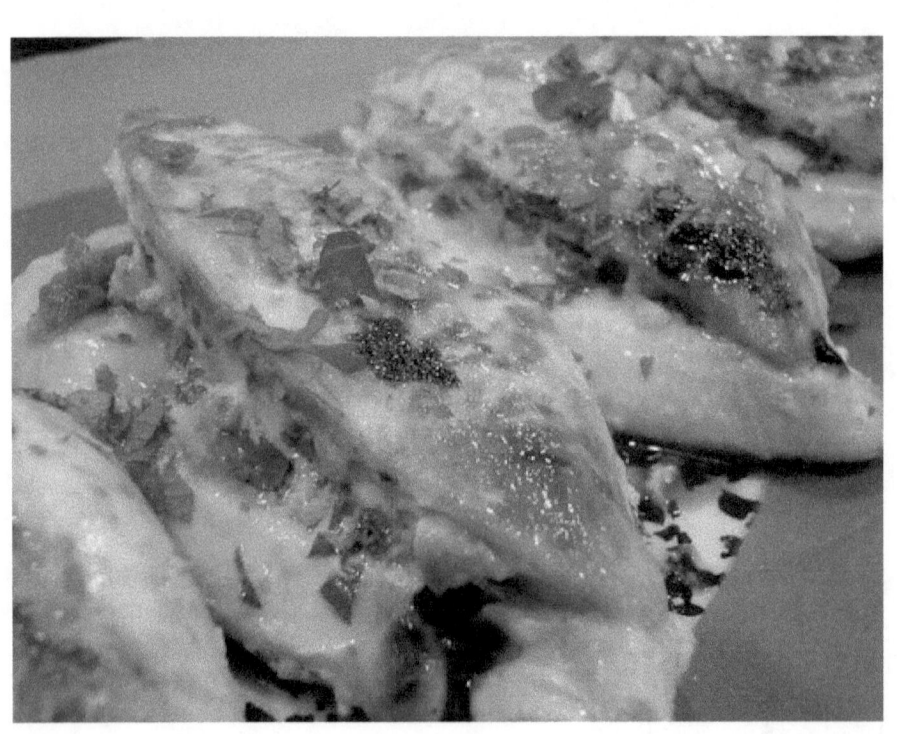

Restaurant-Style Chicken with Yogurt

Cooking Time:
20 minutes

Serve: 4

Ingredients:
1 ¼ lb chicken tenders
1 cup Greek yogurt
1 tbsp lemon juice
1 tbsp fresh dill, chopped For Breading
2 whole eggs, beaten
½ cup breadcrumbs
½ cup all-purpose flour
Salt and black pepper to taste
2 tbsp olive oil

Directions:
1. Preheat air fryer to 380 F. Add breadcrumbs, eggs, and flour in three separate bowls.

2. Season the chicken tenders with salt and pepper and dredge them first into flour, then into eggs, and finally into crumbs.

3. Air Fry them in the fryer for 10 minutes. Flip and cook for 5 more minutes until golden. Mix the yogurt with lemon juice, dill, salt, and pepper until smooth. Serve as a dip to the tenders.

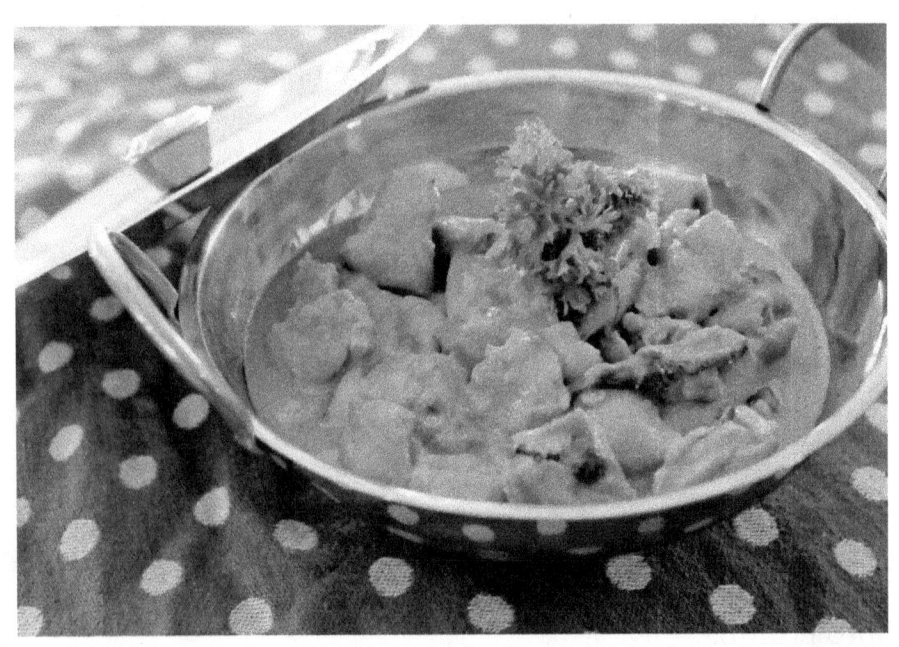

One-Tray Parmesan Chicken Wings

Cooking Time:

20 minutes

Serve:4

Ingredients:

8 chicken wings

1 tsp Dijon mustard Salt to taste

2 tbsp olive oil

2 cloves garlic, crushed

4 tbsp Parmesan cheese, grated

2 tsp fresh parsley, chopped

Directions:

1.Preheat air fryer to 380 F. Grease the frying basket. Season the wings with salt and black pepper. Brush them with mustard.

2.On a plate, pour 2 tbsp of the Parmesan cheese. Coat the wings with Parmesan cheese, drizzle with olive oil, and place in the air fryer basket.

3.AirFry for 15 minutes, turning once. Top with the remaining Parmesan cheese and parsley to serve.

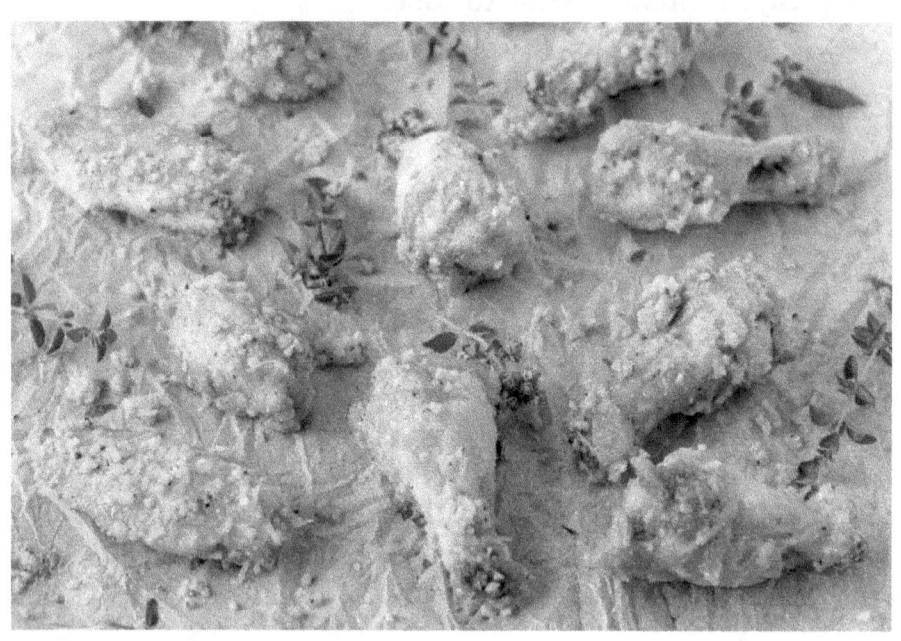

Crunchy Coconut Chicken Dippers

Cooking Time:

20 minutes

Serve: 4

Ingredients:

2 cups coconut flakes

4 chicken breasts, cut into strips

½ cup cornstarch

Salt and black pepper to taste

2 eggs, beaten

Directions:

1. Preheat air fryer to 350 F. Mix salt, pepper, and cornstarch in a bowl. Line a frying basket with parchment paper.

2. Dip the chicken first in the cornstarch, then into the eggs, and finally, coat with coconut flakes.

3. Arrange in the air fryer and Bake for 16 minutes, flipping once until crispy. Serve with berry sauce.

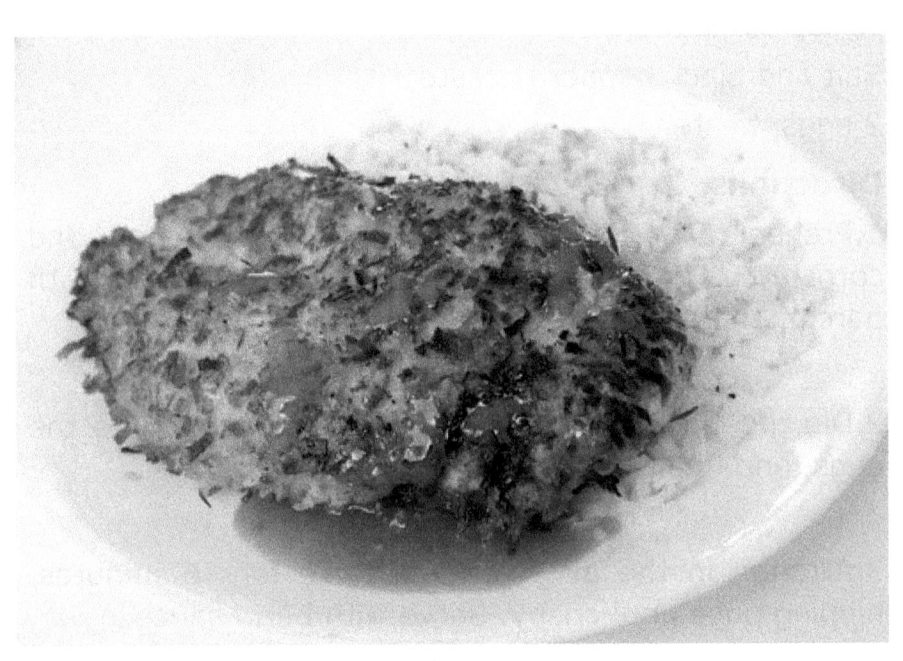

Chicken Fillets with Sweet Chili Adobo

Cooking Time:
20 minutes
Serve:4
Ingredients:

2 chicken breasts, halved

Salt and black pepper to taste

¼ cup sweet chili sauce

1 tsp turmeric

Directions:

1.Preheat air fryer to 390 F. In a bowl, add salt, black pepper, sweet chili sauce, and turmeric; mix well.

2.Lightly brush the chicken with the mixture and place it in the frying basket. Air Fry for 12-14 minutes, turning once halfway through.

3.Serve with a side of steamed greens.

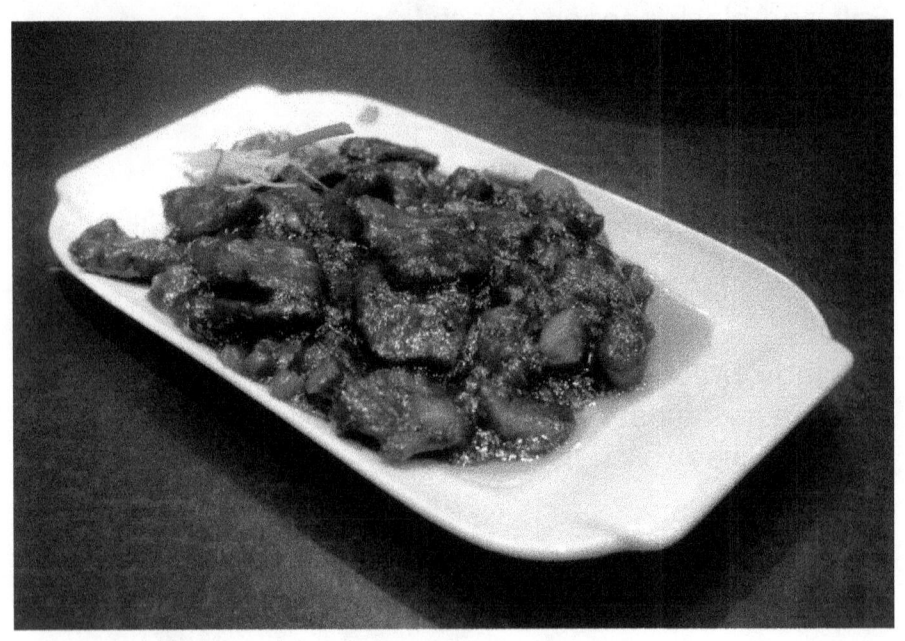

Avocado & Mango Chicken Breasts

Cook Time:

20 minutes

Servings: 2

Ingredients:

2 chicken breasts

1 mango, chopped

1 avocado, sliced

1 red pepper, chopped

1 tbsp balsamic vinegar

2 tbsp olive oil

2 garlic cloves, minced

½ tsp dried oregano

1 tsp mustard powder

Salt and black pepper to taste

Directions:

1. In a bowl, mix garlic, olive oil, and balsamic vinegar. Add in the breasts, cover, and marinate for 2 hours.

2. Preheat the fryer to 360 F. Place the chicken in the frying basket and Air Fry for 12-14 minutes, flipping once. Top with avocado, mango, and red pepper. Drizzle with balsamic vinegar and serve.

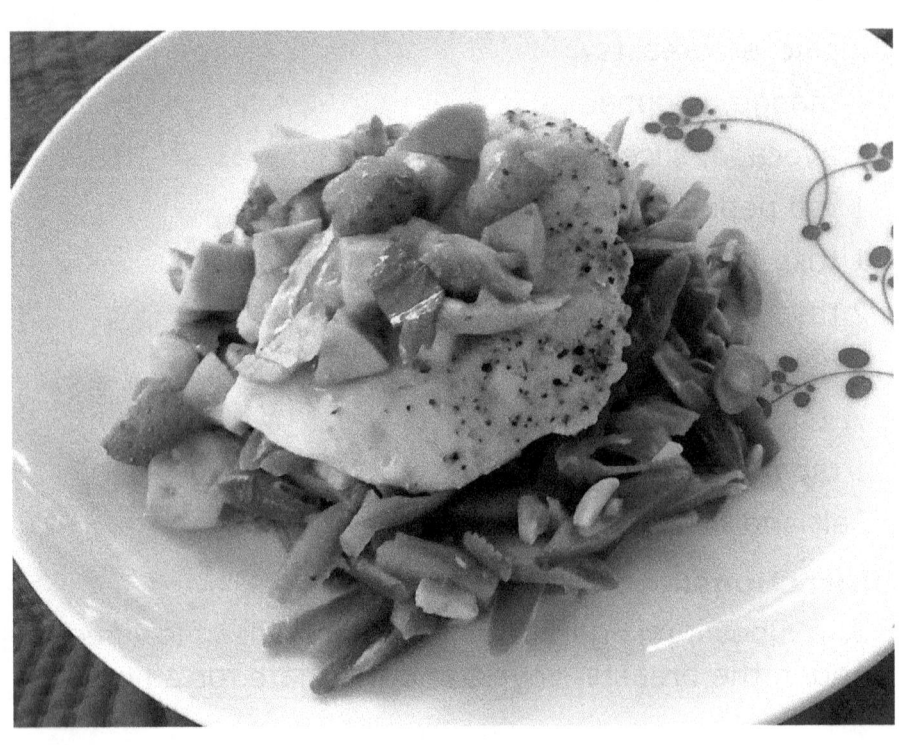

Ham & Cheese Filled Chicken Breasts

Cooking Time:

25 minutes

Serve: 4

Ingredients:

4 chicken breasts

4 ham slices

4 Swiss cheese slices

3 tbsp all-purpose flour

4 tbsp butter

½ tbsp paprika

1 tbsp chicken bouillon granules

¼ cup dry white wine

1 cup heavy whipping cream

Directions:

1. Preheat air fryer to 380 F. Pound the chicken breasts and put a slice of ham and cheese on each one.

2. Fold the edges over the filling and seal them with toothpicks.

3. In a bowl, combine paprika and flour, and coat the chicken. Transfer to the greased air fryer basket and Bake for 15 minutes, turning once.

4. In a large skillet over medium heat, melt the butter and add the bouillon granules, wine, and heavy cream.

5.Bring to a boil, reduce the heat to low, and simmer for 5 minutes. Serve the chicken with sauce.

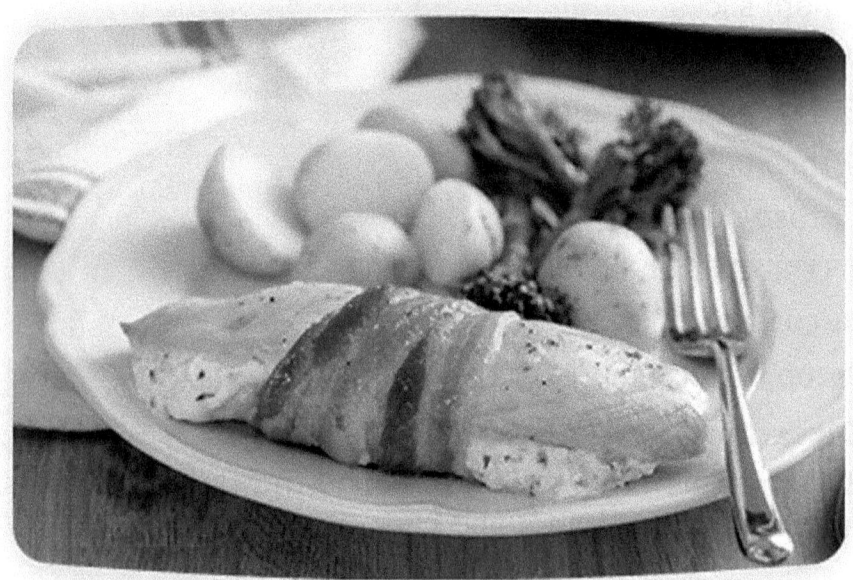

Tasty Chicken Kiev

Cooking Time:

25 minutes

Serve: 4

Ingredients:

1 lb chicken breasts

4 tbsp butter, softened

1 tbsp fresh dill, chopped

2 garlic cloves, minced

1 tbsp lemon juice

Salt and black pepper to taste

1 cup panko breadcrumbs

1 cup plain flour

2 eggs, beaten

Directions:

1. Preheat air fryer to 390 F. In a bowl, mix butter, dill, garlic, lemon juice, salt, and pepper until a smooth paste is formed.

2. Using a sharp knife, make a deep cut of each breast to create a large pocket. Stuff with the butter mixture and secure with toothpicks.

3. Coat the breasts in the flour, then dip in the eggs, and finally in the breadcrumbs. Place chicken in the greased basket and Bake for 8-10 minutes.

4.Turn over and cook for 6 more minutes. Serve sliced.

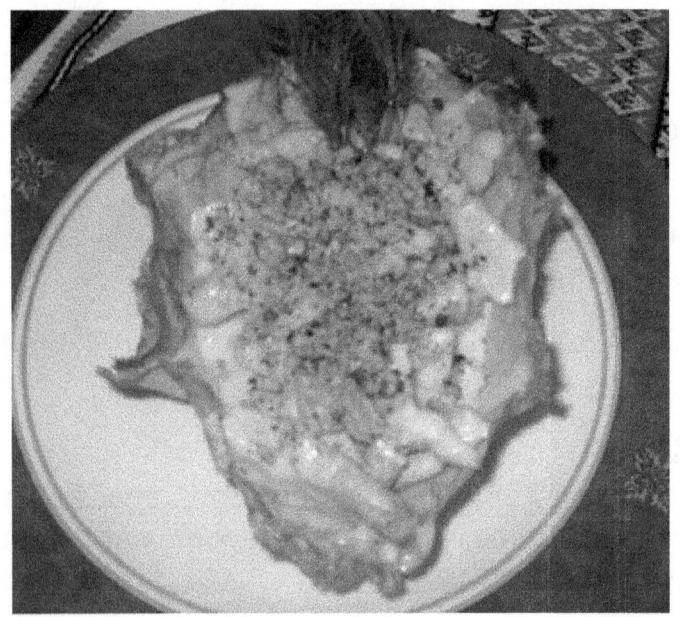

Sweet Mustard Chicken Thighs

Cooking Time:

25 minutes

Serve: 4

Ingredients:

4 chicken thighs, skin-on
1 tbsp honey
1 tsp Dijon mustard
Salt and garlic powder to taste

Directions:

1. In a bowl, mix honey, mustard, garlic powder, and salt.

2. Brush the thighs with the mixture and Air Fry them for 16 minutes at 400 F, turning once halfway through. Serve hot.

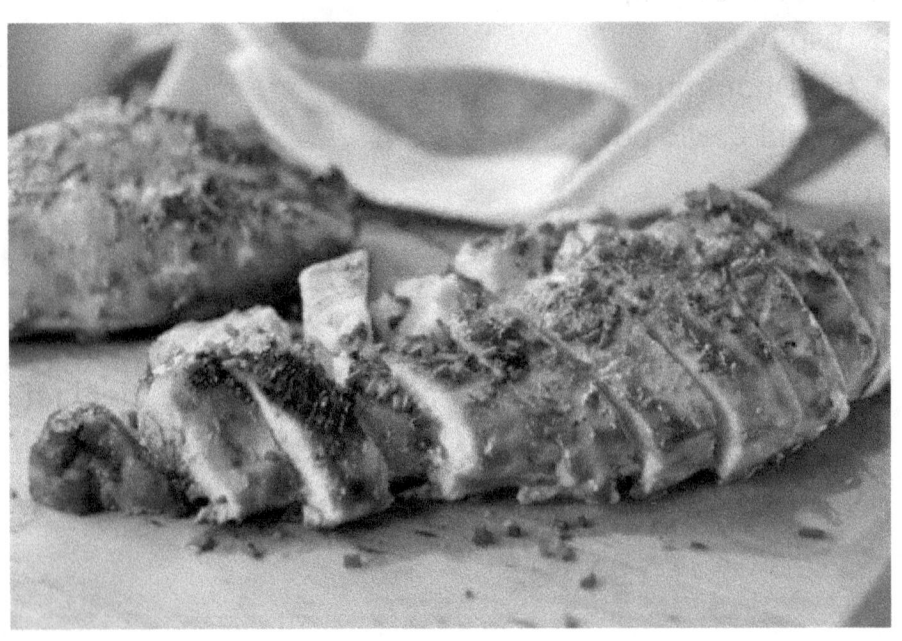

Thyme-Fried Chicken Legs

Cooking Time:

50 minutes

Servings: 4

Ingredients:

4 chicken legs

2 lemons, halved

1 tbsp garlic powder

½ tsp dried oregano

⅓ cup olive oil Salt and black pepper to taste

Directions:

1. Preheat the air fryer to 350 F. Brush the chicken legs with olive oil.

2. Sprinkle with lemon juice and arrange in the frying basket. In a bowl, mix oregano, garlic powder, salt, and pepper.

3. Scatter the seasoning mixture over the chicken and Bake the legs in the air fryer for 14-16 minutes, shaking once.

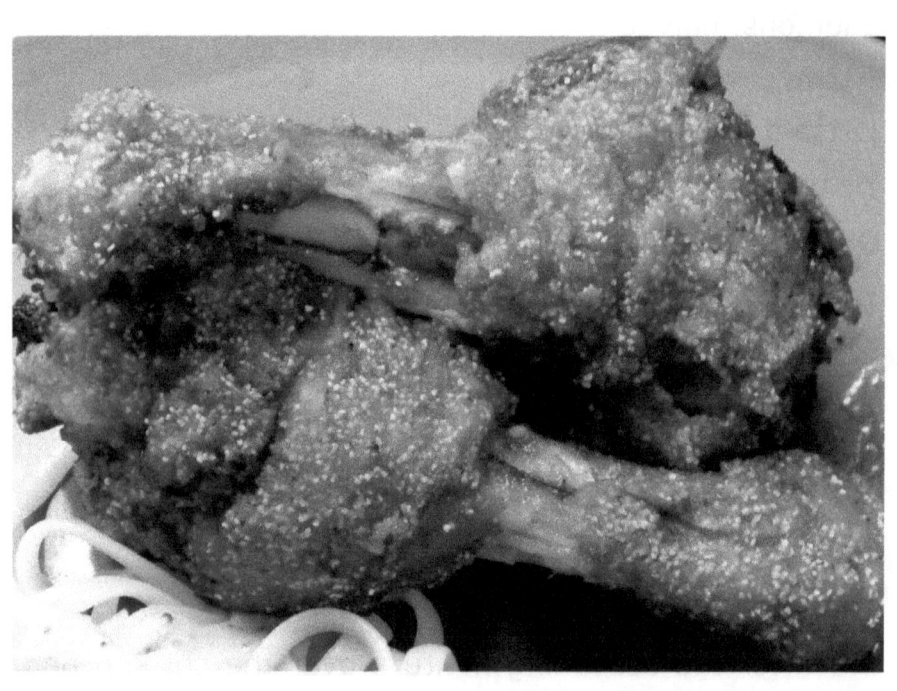

Honey-Glazed Turkey

Cooking Time:

50 minutes

Servings:4

Ingredients:

1½ lb turkey tenderloins

¼ cup honey

2 tbsp Dijon mustard

½ tsp dried thyme

½ tsp garlic powder

½ onion powder

1 tbsp olive oil

½ tbsp spicy brown mustard

Salt and black pepper to taste

Directions:

1. Preheat air fryer to 375°F. Combine the honey, mustard, thyme, garlic powder, and onion powder in a bowl to make a paste.

2. Season the turkey with salt and pepper, then spread the honey paste all over it.

3. Put the turkey in the fryer basket and spray with olive oil, then air fry for 15 minutes. Turn it over and spray again before frying for 10-15 more minutes.

4. Remove the turkey, cover loosely with foil and let stand 10 minutes before slicing. Serve and enjoy!

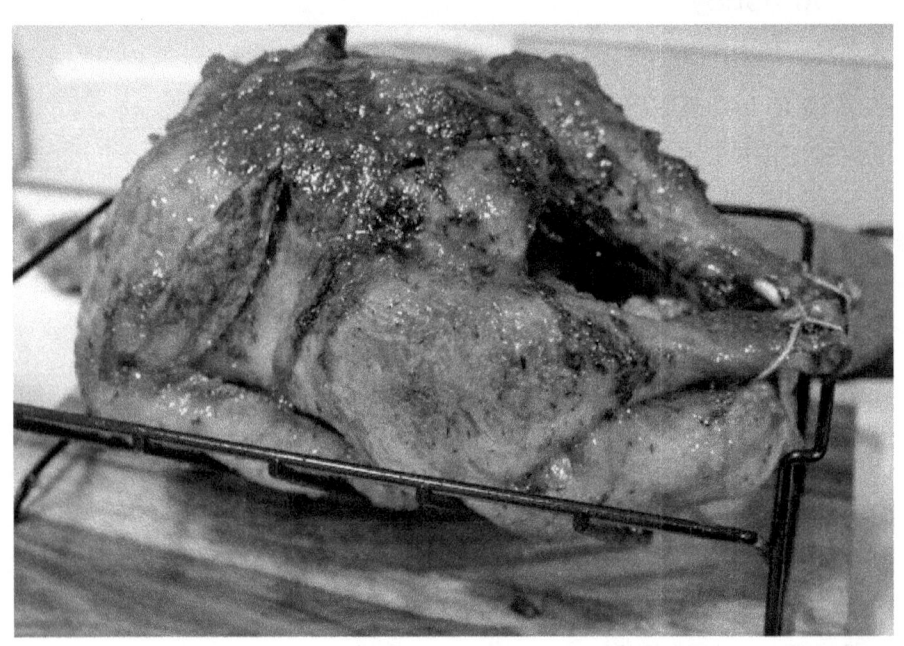

Spice-Rubbed Jerk Chicken Wings

Cook Time:
25 minutes
Servings: 4
Ingredients:

1 lb chicken wings
2 tbsp olive oil
3 cloves garlic, minced
1 tbsp chili powder
½ tbsp cinnamon powder
½ tsp allspice
1 habanero pepper, seeded
1 tbsp soy sauce
½ tbsp lemon pepper
¼ cup red wine vinegar
3 tbsp lime juice
½ tbsp grated ginger
½ tbsp fresh thyme, chopped
⅓ tbsp sugar

Directions:

1. In a bowl, add olive oil, soy sauce, garlic, habanero pepper, allspice, cinnamon powder, chili powder, lemon pepper, sugar, thyme, ginger, lime juice, and red wine vinegar; mix well.

2. Add the chicken wings to the mixture and toss to coat. Cover and refrigerate for 1 hour.

3.Preheat air fryer to 380 F. Remove the chicken from the fridge, drain all the liquid, and pat dry with paper towels.

4.Working in batches, cook the wings in the air fryer for 16 minutes in total. Shake once halfway through. Remove to a serving platter and serve with a blue cheese dip or ranch dressing.

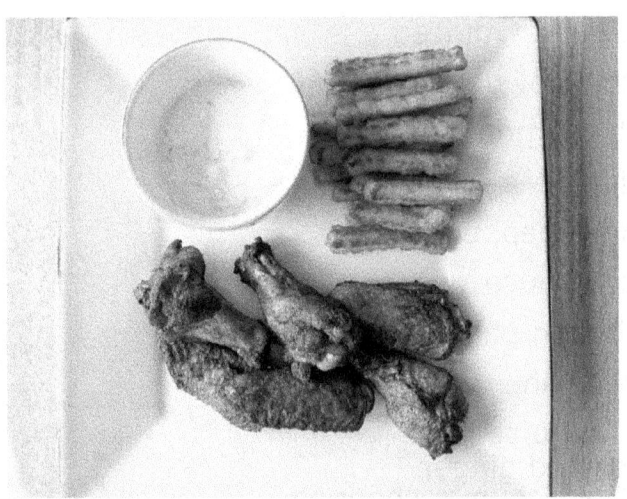

Sweet Sesame Chicken Wings

Cooking Time:

25 minutes

Servings:4

Ingredients:

1 lb chicken wings

2 tbsp sesame oil

1 tbsp maple syrup

Salt and black pepper to taste

3 tbsp sesame seeds

Directions:

1.In a bowl, add wings, sesame oil, maple syrup, salt, and pepper and stir to coat. In another bowl, add the sesame seeds and roll up the wings in the seeds.

2.Arrange the wings in an even layer inside your air fryer and cook for 12 minutes at 360 F, turning once halfway through. Serve.

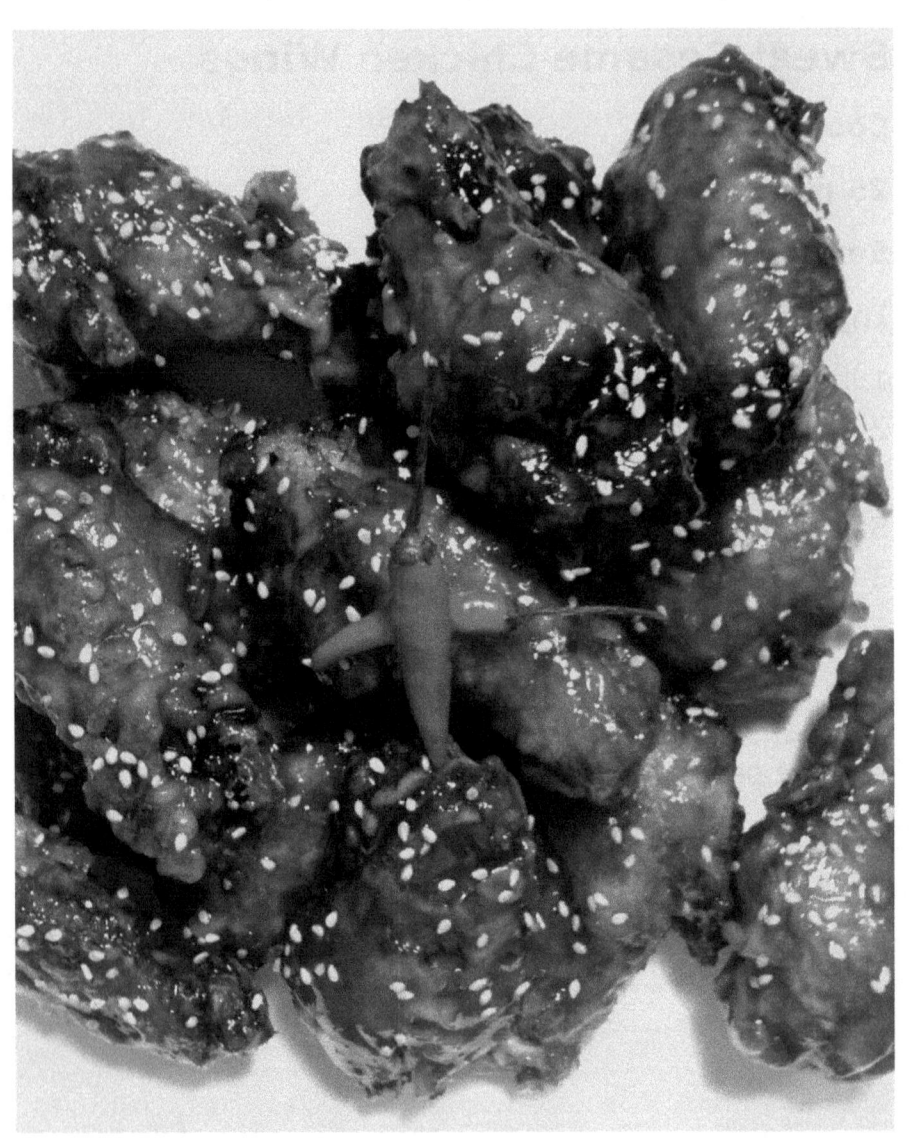

Crispy Breaded Chicken Breasts

Cooking Time:

20 minutes

Servings: 4

Ingredients:

4 chicken breasts, sliced

1 tbsp Worcestershire sauce

¼ cup onions, chopped

1 tbsp brown sugar

¼ cup yellow mustard

½ cup ketchup

Directions:

1. Preheat air fryer to 360 F. In a bowl, mix sugar, 1 cup of water, ketchup, onions, mustard, Worcestershire sauce, and salt.

2. Place the chicken into the mixture and let marinate for 10 minutes. Transfer the chicken to the frying basket and Air Fry for 15 minutes, flipping once. Serve with the sauce.

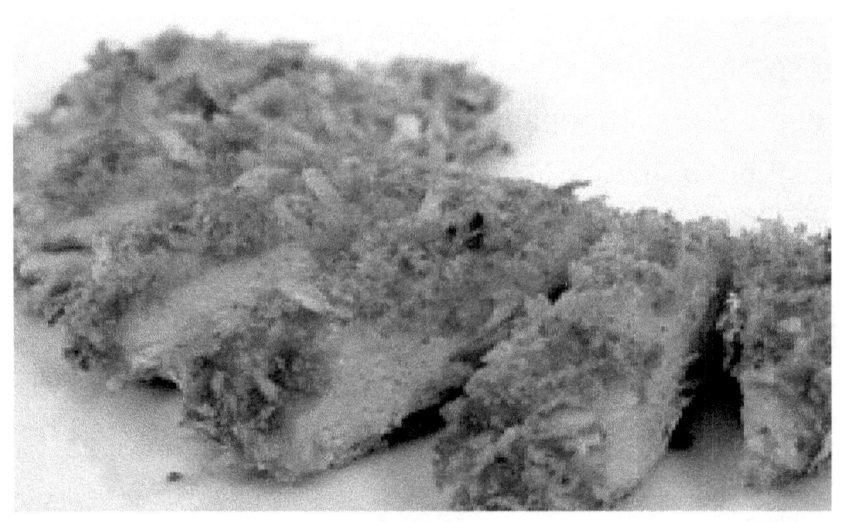

Crispy Chicken Tenderloins

Cooking Time:

15 minutes

Servings: 4

Ingredients:

8 chicken tenderloins

2 tbsp butter, melted

1 cup seasoned breadcrumbs

DIRECTIONS

1. Preheat air fryer to 380 F. Dip the chicken in the eggs, then coat with the seasoned crumbs.

2. Coat the air fryer basket with some butter and place in the chicken.

3. Brush with the remaining butter and cook for 14-16 minutes, shaking once halfway through. Serve with your favorite dip.

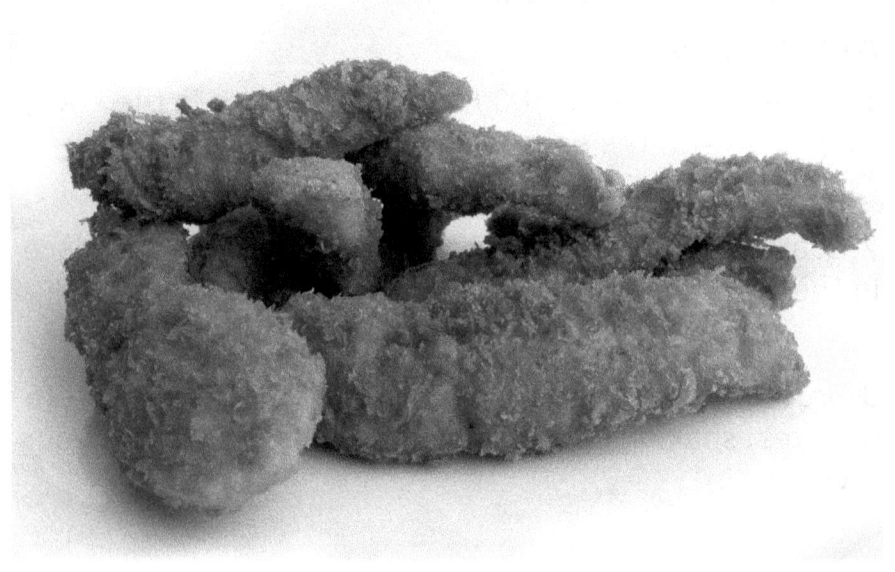

Gluten-Free Crunchy Chicken

Cooking Time:

25 minutes

Servings:4

Ingredients:

2 garlic cloves, minced

1 lb chicken breasts, sliced

½ tsp dried thyme

1 cup potato flakes

Salt and black pepper to taste

½ cup cheddar cheese, grated

½ cup mayonnaise

1 lemon, zested

Directions:

1.Preheat air fryer to 350 F. In a bowl, mix garlic, potato flakes, cheddar cheese, thyme, lemon zest, salt, and pepper.

2.Brush the chicken with mayonnaise, then roll in the potato mixture.

3.Place in the greased air fryer basket and Air Fry for 18-20 minutes, shaking once halfway through. Serve warm.

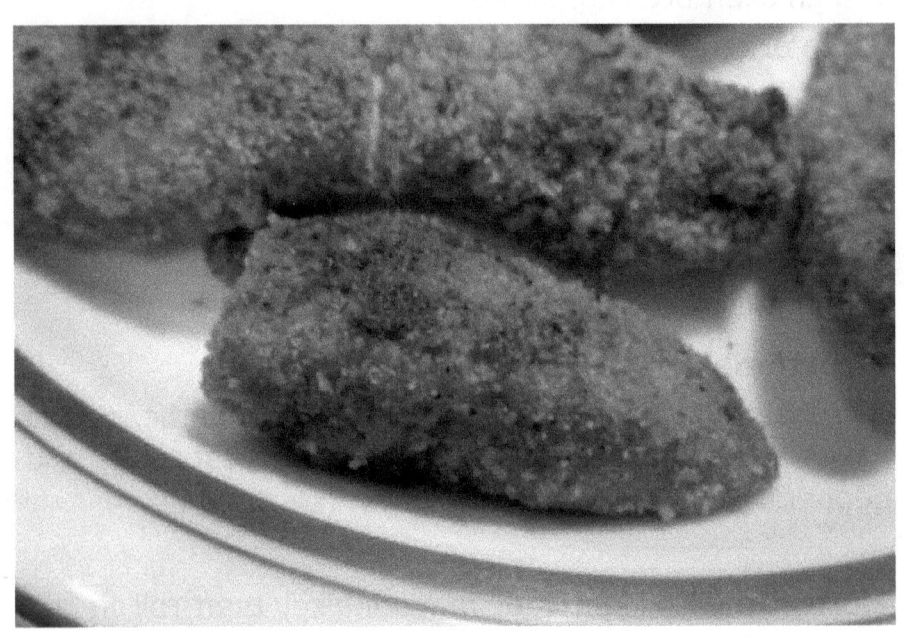

Gingery Chicken Wings

Cooking Time:
25 minutes
Servings: 4
Ingredients:
8 chicken drumsticks

1 tbsp olive oil

1 tbsp sesame oil

1 tbsp honey

3 tbsp light soy sauce

2 crushed garlic clove

1 small knob fresh ginger, grated

2 tbsp black sesame seeds, toasted

Directions:

1. Preheat air fryer to 400 F. Add all ingredients to a freezer bag, except for sesame seeds.

2. Seal up and massage until the drumsticks are well coated. Place the drumsticks in the basket and cook for 10 minutes.

3. Flip and cook for 10 more minutes. Sprinkle with sesame seeds and serve.

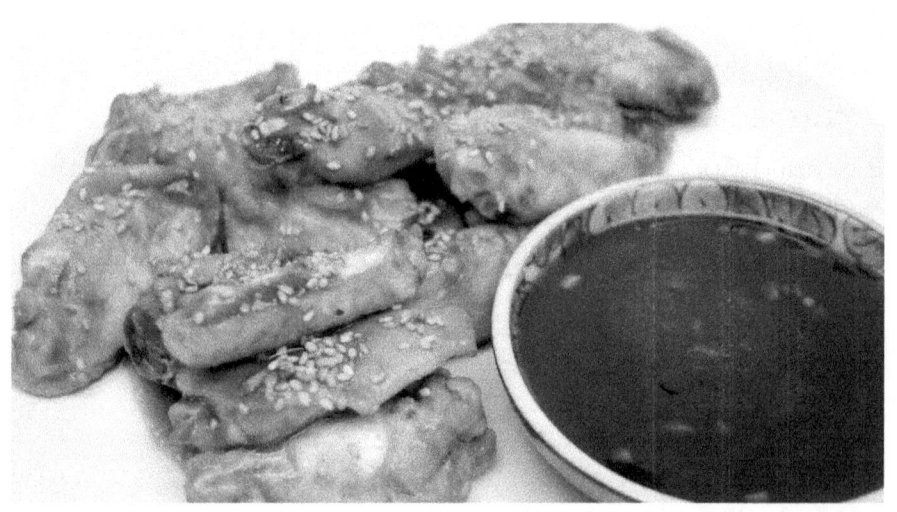

Rosemary & Oyster Chicken Breasts

Cook Time:

25 minutes

Servings: 2

Ingredients:

2 chicken breasts

1 tbsp ginger paste

2 fresh rosemary sprigs, chopped

2 lemon wedges

1 tbsp soy sauce

1 tbsp olive oil

1 tbsp oyster sauce

1 tbsp brown sugar

Directions:

1. Add ginger, soy sauce, and olive oil in a bowl. Add in the chicken and mix to coat well.

2. Cover the bowl and refrigerate for 30 minutes. Preheat air fryer to 370 F. Transfer the marinated chicken to a baking dish and Bake in the fryer for 6 minutes.

3. Mix oyster sauce, rosemary, and brown sugar in a bowl. Pour the sauce over the chicken. Return to the air fryer and Bake for 10 minutes.

4. Remove the rosemary and serve with lemon wedges.

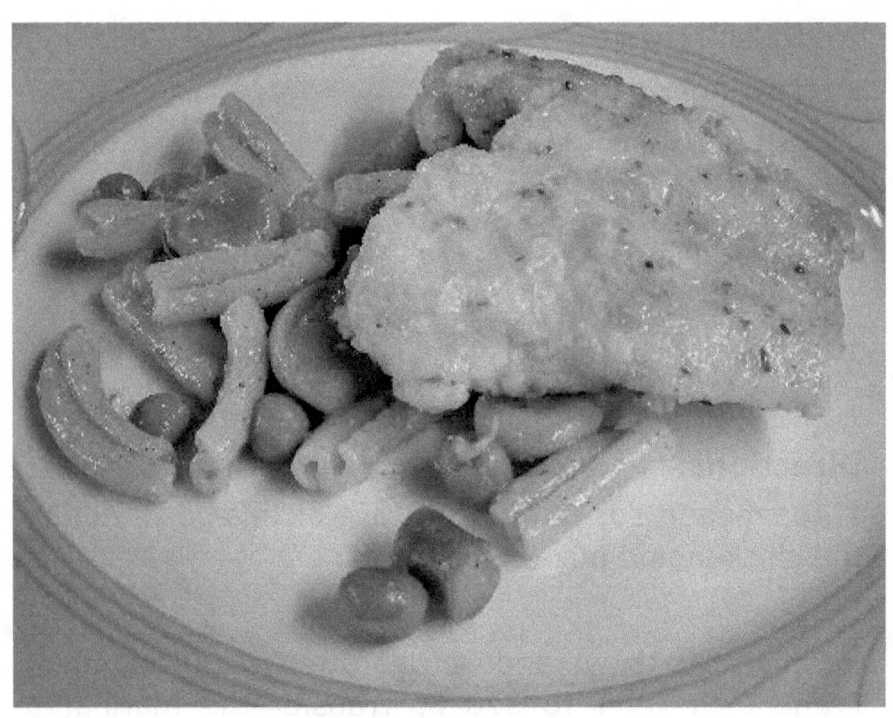

Chicken Thighs with Parmesan Crust

Cooking Time:

25 minutes

Servings: 4

Ingredients:

½ cup Italian breadcrumbs

2 tbsp Parmesan cheese, grated

1 tbsp butter, melted

4 chicken thighs

½ cup marinara sauce

½ cup Monterrey jack cheese, shredded

Directions:

1. Preheat air fryer to 380 F. In a bowl, mix the crumbs with Parmesan cheese.

2. Brush the thighs with butter. Dip each thigh into the crumb mixture. Arrange them on the greased air fryer basket.

3. Air Fry for 6-7 minutes at 380 F, flip, top with marinara sauce and shredded Monterrey Jack cheese, and continue to cook for another 4-5 minutes. Serve immediately

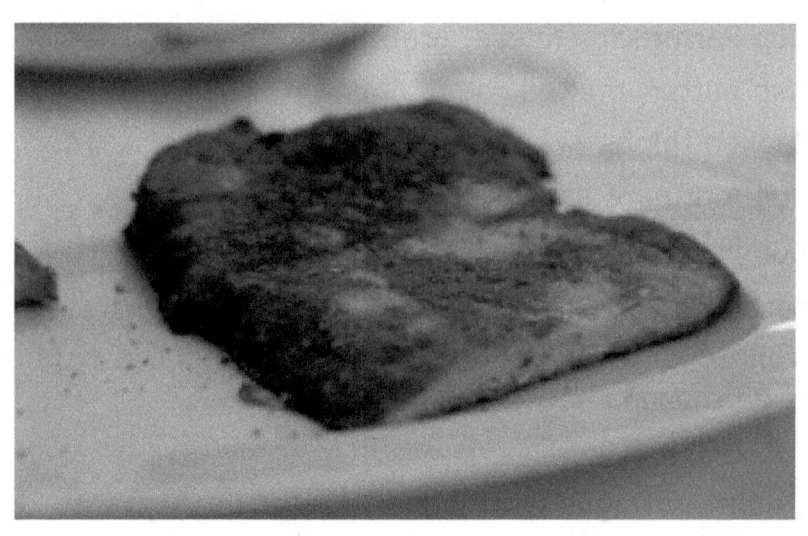

Chicken & Baby Potato Traybake

Cooking Time:

20 minutes

Servings: 4

Ingredients:

1 lb chicken drumsticks, skin on and bone-in

3 shallots, quartered

Salt and black pepper to taste

1 tbsp cayenne pepper

1 lb baby potatoes, halved

½ tsp garlic powder

2 tbsp olive oil

1 cup cherry tomatoes

Directions:

1. Preheat air fryer to 360 F. Place the chicken in a baking tray and add in shallots, potatoes, oil, garlic powder, salt, and pepper; toss to coat.

2. Place the tray in the fryer and Bake for 18-20 minutes, shaking once. Slide the basket out and add in the cherry tomatoes. Cook for another 5 minutes until charred.

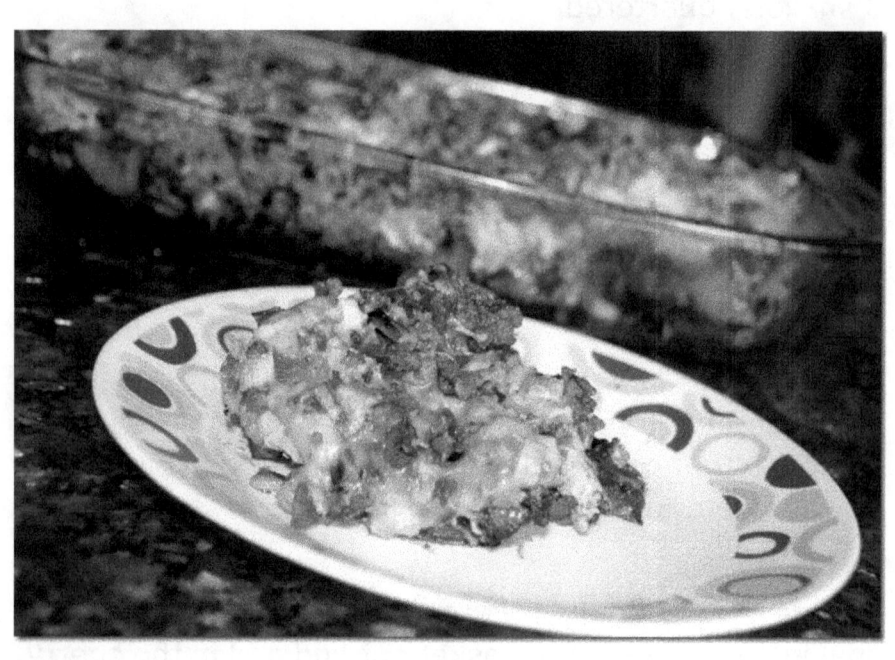

Portuguese Roasted Whole Chicken

Cook Time:
50 minutes
Servings: 4
Ingredients:

1 3 lb whole chicken
1 lime, juiced
Portuguese seasoning:
Salt and black pepper to taste
1 tsp chili powder
1 tsp garlic powder
1 tsp oregano
1 tsp ground coriander
1 tsp cumin
2 tbsp olive oil
1 tsp paprika

Directions:

1. In a bowl, pour oregano, garlic powder, chili powder, coriander, paprika, cumin, black pepper, salt, and olive oil and mix well.

2. Rub onto the chicken and refrigerate the chicken for 20 minutes to marinate. Preheat air fryer to 350 F.

3. Remove the chicken from the fridge, place it breast side down in the greased frying basket, and Bake for 30 minutes.

4.After, flip the chicken breast-side up and continue cooking for 10-15 minutes. When over, let it rest for 10 minutes, then drizzle with lime juice and serve.

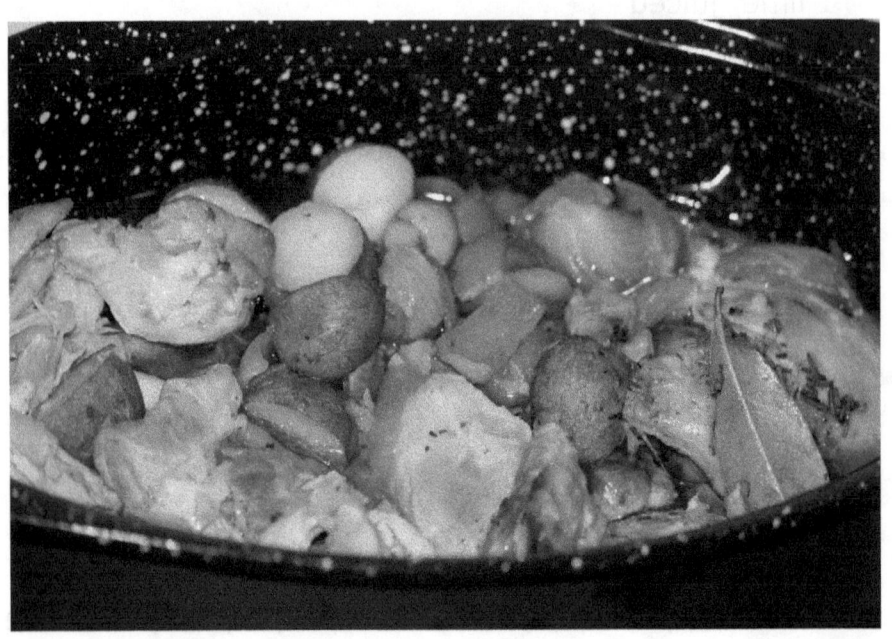

Turkey & Veggie Skewers

Cooking Time:

20 minutes

Servings: 4

Ingredients:

1 lb turkey breast, cubed

2 tbsp fresh rosemary, chopped

Salt and black pepper to taste

1 green bell pepper, cut into chunks

1 red bell pepper, cut into chunks

1 cup cherry tomatoes

1 red onion, cut into wedges

Directions:

1. Preheat air fryer to 350 F. Spray the air fryer basket with cooking spray. In a bowl, mix the turkey, salt, and black pepper.

2. Thread the vegetables and turkey cubes alternately onto skewers. Spray with cooking spray and transfer to the frying basket. Bake for 15 minutes, flipping once halfway through. Serve sprinkled with fresh rosemary.

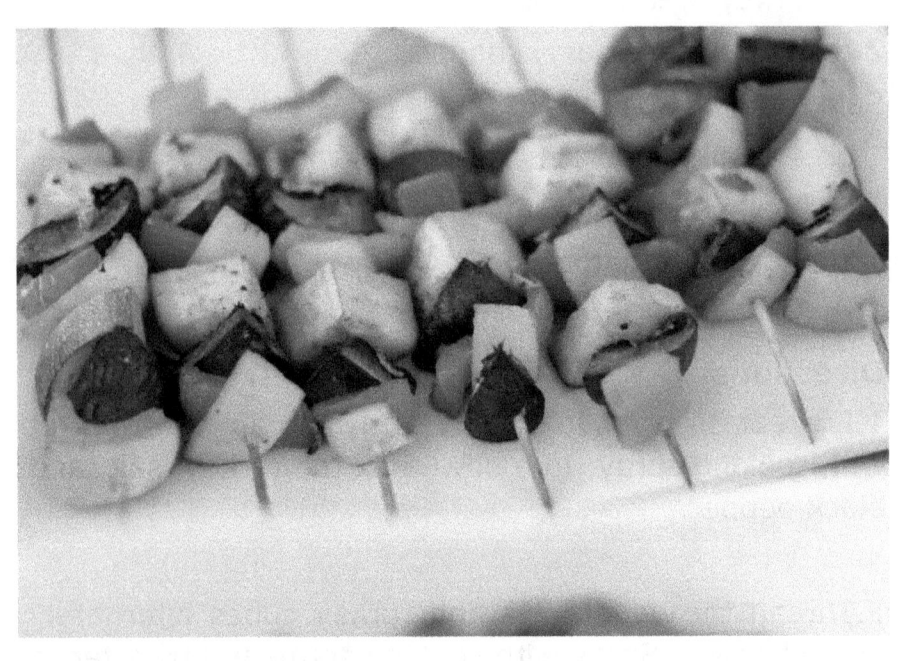

Chipotle Buttered Turkey

Cooking Time:

25 minutes

Servings: 4

Ingredients:

1 lb turkey breast, sliced

2 cups panko breadcrumbs

½ tsp chipotle chili pepper

Salt and black pepper to taste

1 stick butter, melted

DIRECTIONS

1. In a bowl, combine panko and chipotle chili pepper. Sprinkle turkey with salt and black pepper, and brush with some butter.

2. Coat the turkey with the panko mixture. Transfer to the frying basket dish and top with butter.

3. Air Fry for 10 minutes at 390 F. Shake, drizzle the remaining butter, and Bake for 5 more minutes, until nice and crispy. Serve with enchilada sauce.

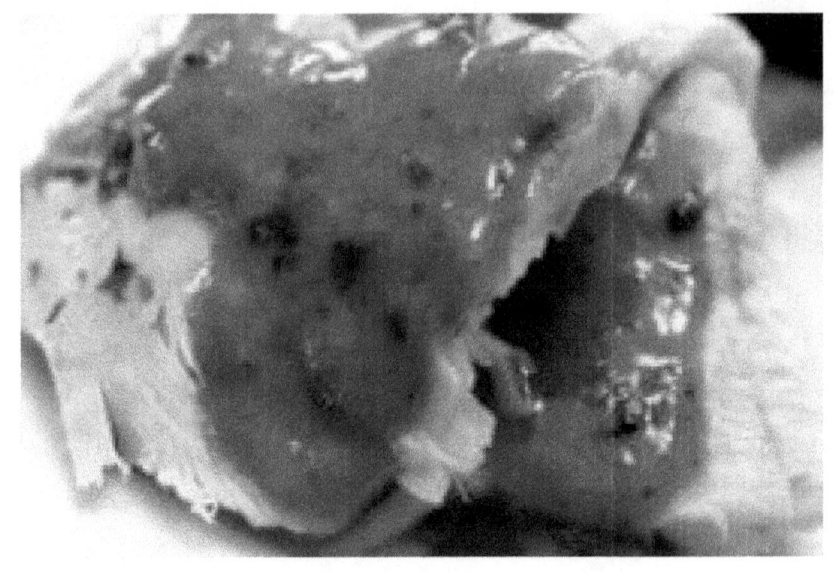

Sweet Curried Chicken Cutlets

Cook Time:
35 minutes
Servings:4
Ingredients:

1lb chicken breasts, halved crosswise
2 tbsp garlic mayonnaise
½ tsp chili powder
½ tsp curry powder
½ tsp brown sugar
2 tbsp soy sauce

Directions:

1.Put the chicken halves between 2 pieces of plastic wrap and gently pound them to ¼-inch thickness using a rolling pin.

2.In a bowl, mix in soy sauce, brown sugar, curry powder, and chili powder. Add in the chicken and toss to coat.

3.Cover with plastic wrap and refrigerate for 1 hour. Preheat air fryer to 350 F.

4.Remove the chicken from the marinade and place it in the greased frying basket. Air Fry for 8 minutes, flip, and cook further for 6 more minutes. Serve with garlic mayonnaise.

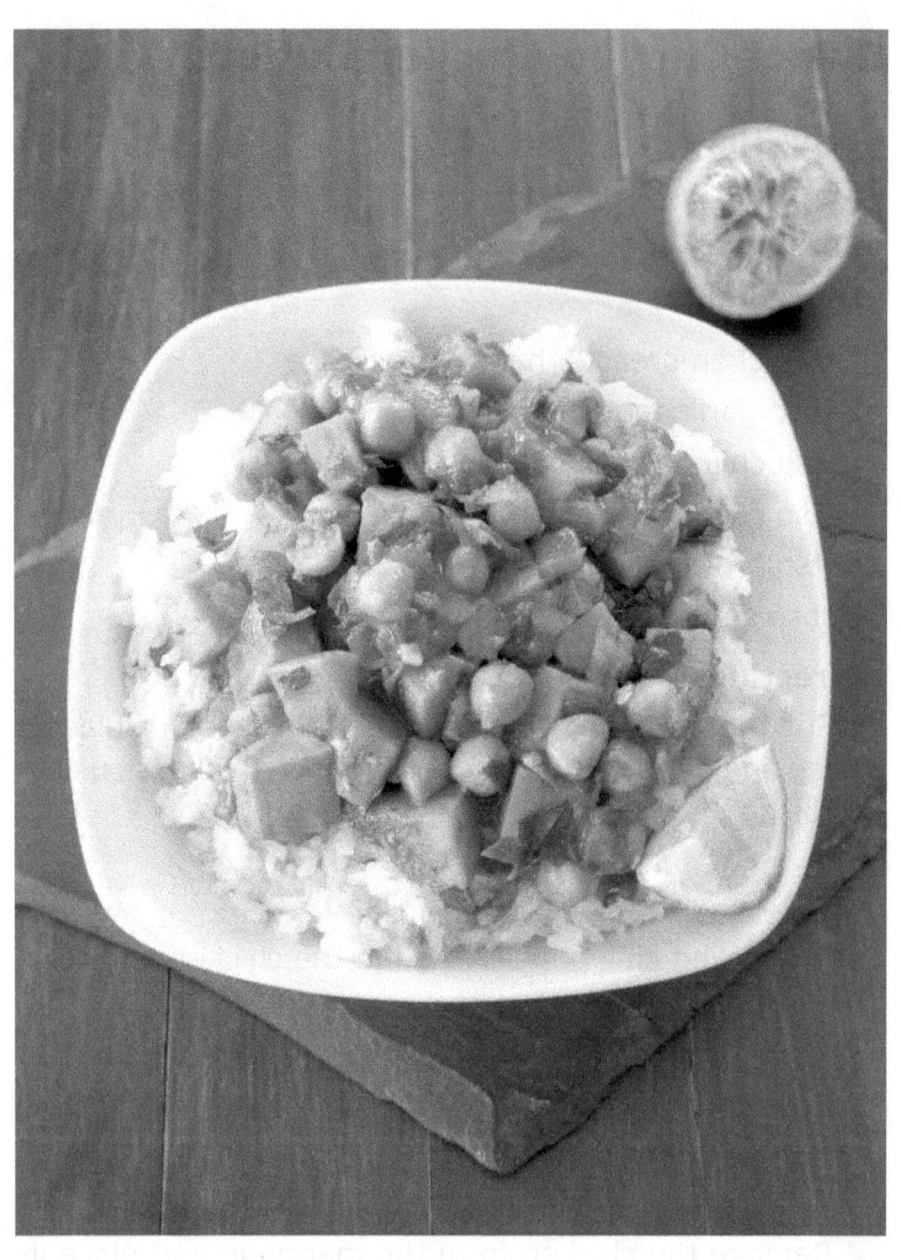

Chicken Thighs with Herby Tomatoes

Cooking Time:

25 minutes

Servings: 2

Ingredients:

1 chicken thighs

2 ripe tomatoes, sliced

2 cloves garlic, minced

¼ tbsp dried tarragon

¼ tbsp olive oil

¼ tsp red pepper flakes

Salt and black pepper to taste

Directions:

1. Preheat air fryer to 390 F. Add the tomatoes, red pepper flakes, tarragon, garlic, and olive oil to a bowl. Mix well.

2. Season the chicken with salt and pepper and place in a greased baking dish. Bake in the fryer for 14 minutes, flipping once. Top with tomato mixture and Bake for 5 more minutes. Serve warm.

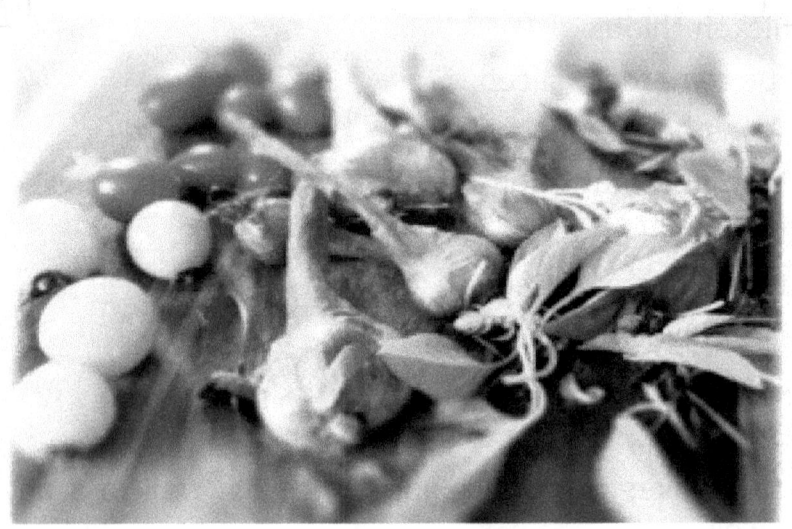

BBQ Whole Chicken

Cooking Time:

35 minutes

Servings: 3

Ingredients:

1 whole small chicken, cut into pieces
Salt to taste
½ tsp smoked paprika
½ tsp garlic powder
1 cup BBQ sauce

Directions:

1. Mix salt, paprika, and garlic powder and coat the chicken pieces. Place in the air fryer basket and Bake for 18 minutes at 400 F.

2. Remove to a plate and brush with barbecue sauce. Wipe the fryer clean from the chicken fat. Return the chicken to the fryer, skin-side up, and Bake for 5 more minutes at 340 F.

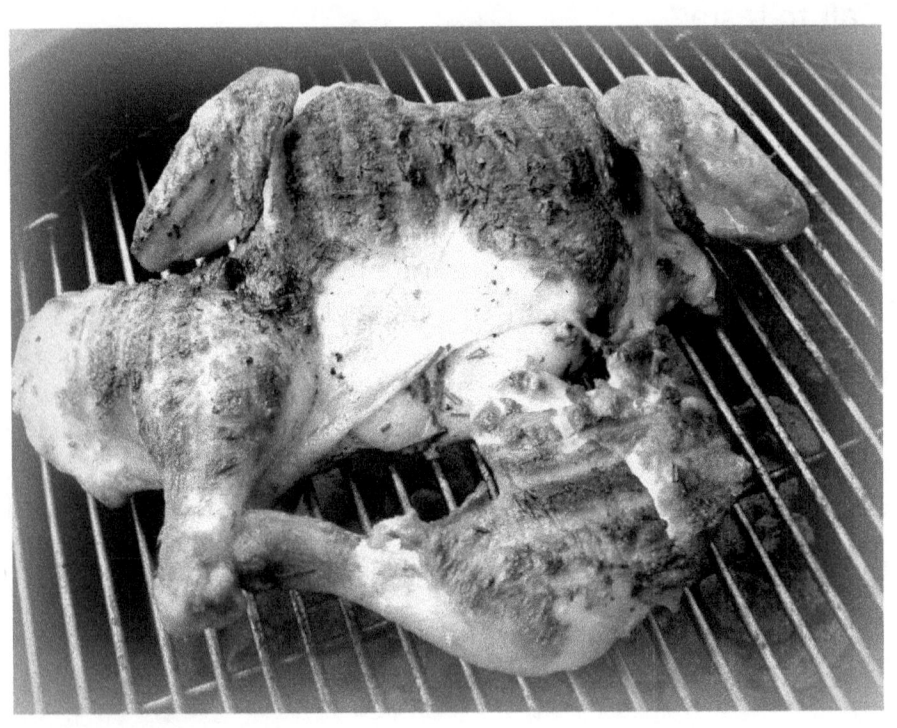

Thyme Turkey Nuggets

Cooking Time:

20 minutes

Servings: 2

Ingredients:

½ lb ground turkey
1 egg, beaten
1 cup breadcrumbs
½ tsp dried thyme
½ tsp fresh parsley, chopped
Salt and black pepper to taste

Directions:

1. Preheat air fryer to 350 F. In a bowl, mix ground turkey, thyme, parsley, salt, and pepper. Shape the mixture into balls.

2. Dip in the breadcrumbs, then in egg, and in the crumbs again. Place the nuggets in the air fryer basket, spray with cooking spray and Air Fry for 12-14 minutes, shaking once. Serve hot.

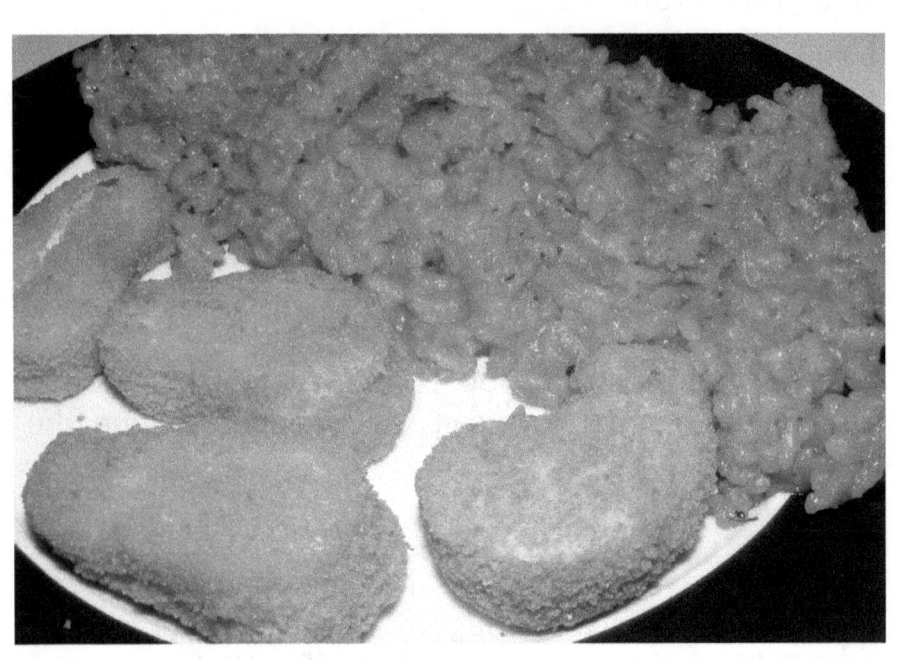

Hot Chili Chicken Wings

Cook Time:
25 minutes
Servings: 2
Ingredients:

8 chicken wings
1 cup corn flour
½ cup white wine
1 tsp chili paste
1-inch fresh ginger, grated
1 tbsp olive oil

Directions:

1. Preheat air fryer to 360 F. In a bowl, mix ginger, chili paste, and wine.

2. Add in the chicken wings and marinate for 30 minutes.

3. Remove the chicken, drain, and coat with corn flour. Brush with olive oil and place in the frying basket.

4. Air Fry for 14-16 minutes, shaking once until crispy on the outside. Serve

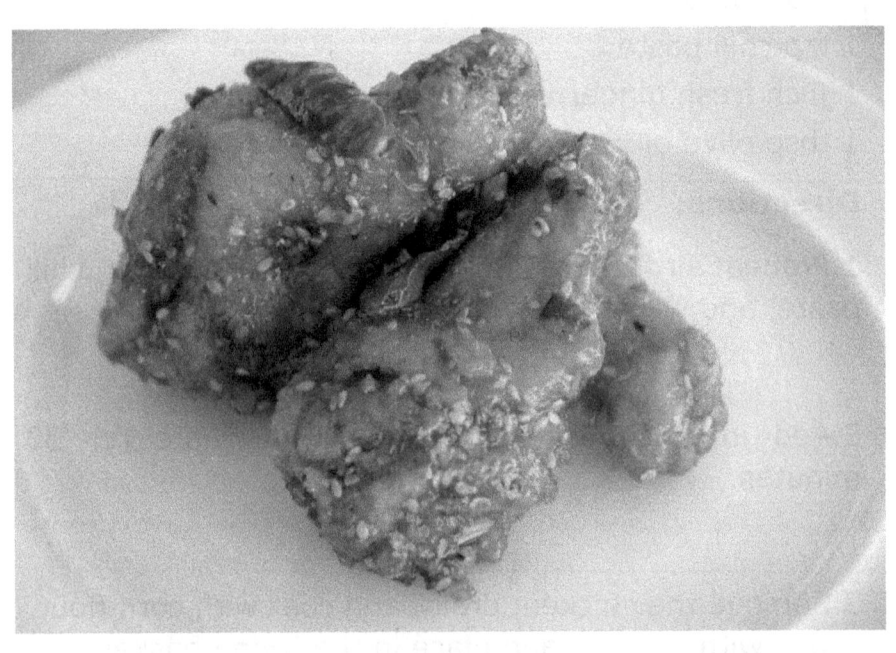

Homemade Chicken Patties

Cooking Time:

20 minutes

Servings: 4

Ingredients:

1 lb ground chicken

½ onion, chopped

2 garlic cloves, chopped

1 egg, beaten

½ cup breadcrumbs

½ tsp cumin

½ tbsp paprika

½ tbsp coriander seeds, crushed

Salt and black pepper to taste

Directions:

1. In a bowl, mix chicken, onion, garlic, egg, breadcrumbs, cumin, paprika, coriander, salt, and black pepper.

2. Use your hands to shape into 4 patties. Arrange on the greased air fryer basket and Bake for 10-12 minutes at 380 F, turning once halfway through. Serve and enjoy!

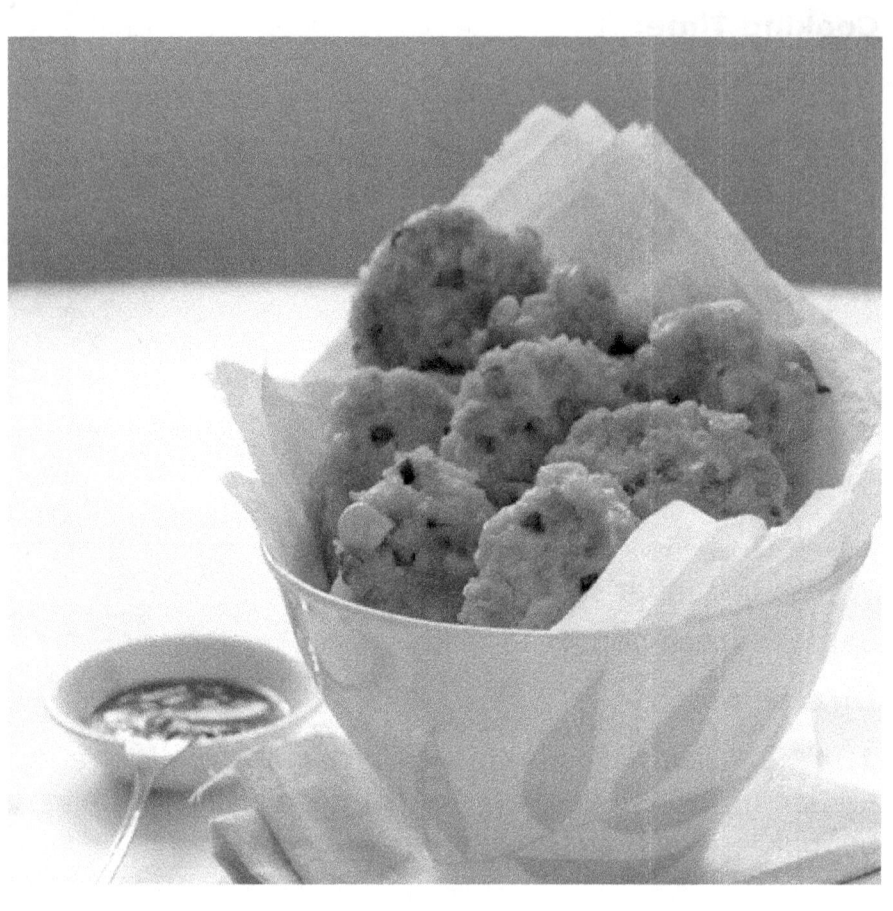

Chicken Pinchos with Salsa Verde

Cooking Time:

35 minutes

Servings: 4

Ingredients:

4 chicken breasts, cut into large cubes

Salt to taste

1 tsp chili powder

1 tbsp maple syrup

½ cup soy sauce

2 red peppers, cut into sticks

1 green pepper, cut into sticks

8 mushrooms, halved

2 tbsp sesame seeds

Salsa Verde:

1 garlic clove

2 tbsp olive oil

Zest and juice from 1 lime

¼ cup fresh parsley, chopped

A bunch of skewers

Directions:

1. In a bowl, mix chili powder, salt, maple syrup, soy sauce, and sesame seeds and toss in the chicken to coat.

2. Start stacking up the ingredients, alternately, on skewers: red pepper, green pepper, a chicken cube, and a mushroom half, until the skewer is fully loaded.

Repeat the process for all the ingredients.

3. Preheat air fryer to 330 F. Brush the pinchos with soy sauce mixture and place them into the frying basket.

4. Grease with cooking spray and cook for 20 minutes, flipping once halfway through. Blend all the salsa verde ingredients in a food processor until you obtain a chunky paste.

5. Taste and adjust the seasoning with salt. Arrange the pinchos on a platter and serve with the salsa verde. Enjoy!

Juicy Chicken Fillets with Peppers

Cooking Time:

35 minutes

Servings: 2

Ingredients:

2 chicken fillets, cubed

Salt and black pepper to taste

1 cup flour

2 eggs

½ cup apple cider vinegar

½ tbsp ginger paste

½ tbsp garlic paste

1 tbsp sugar

1 red chili, minced

2 tbsp tomato puree

1 red bell pepper, seeded, cut into strips

1 green bell pepper, seeded, cut into strips

1 tbsp paprika

4 tbsp water

Directions:

1. Preheat air fryer to 350 F. Pour the flour in a bowl, add in eggs, salt, and black pepper and whisk.

2. Put chicken cubes in the flour mixture; mix to coat and place them in the frying basket. Spray with cooking

spray and Air Fry for 8 minutes.

3.Shake the basket, and cook for 7 more minutes until golden and crispy.

4.In a bowl, add water, apple cider vinegar, sugar, ginger paste, garlic paste, red chili, tomato puree, and paprika; mix with a fork.

5.Place a skillet over medium heat and spray with cooking spray. Add the red and green pepper strips. Stir and cook until the peppers are sweaty but still crunchy.

6.Pour the chili mixture over, stir, and simmer for 10 minutes. Serve the chicken drizzled with pepper-chili sauce.

Crumbed Sage Chicken Scallopini

Cooking Time:

12 minutes

Serve: 2

Ingredients:

4 chicken breasts

3 oz breadcrumbs

2 tbsp Parmesan cheese, grated

2 oz flour

2 eggs, beaten

1 tbsp fresh sage, chopped

1 lemon, cut into wedges

Directions:

1. Preheat air fryer to 370 F. Place some plastic wrap underneath and on top of the breasts. Using a rolling pin, beat the meat until it becomes skinny.

2. In a bowl, combine Parmesan cheese, sage, and breadcrumbs. Dip the chicken in the egg first, and then in the flour.

3. Spray with cooking spray and Air Fry for 14-16 minutes, flipping once halfway through. Serve with lemon wedges.

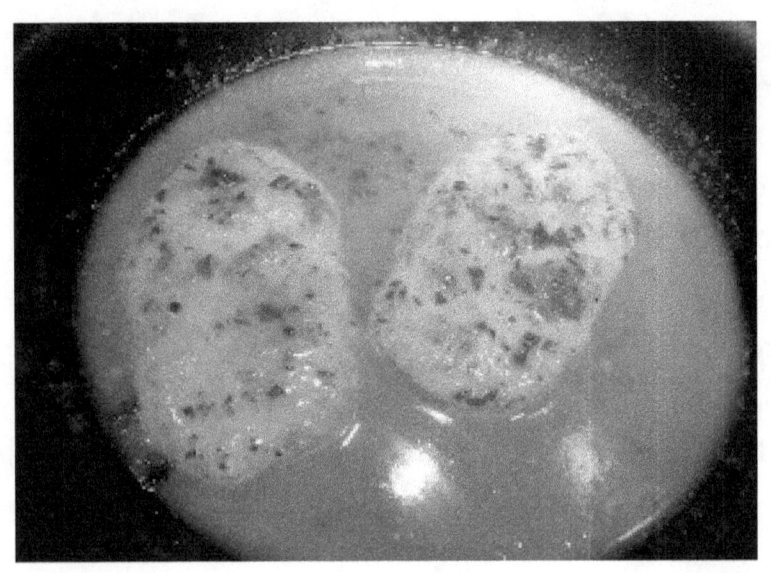

Hawaiian-Style Chicken

Cook Time:
20 minutes
Servings:4
Ingredients:

4 chicken breasts, cubed
2 garlic cloves, minced
½ cup ketchup
½ tbsp ginger, minced
½ cup soy sauce
2 tbsp sherry
½ cup pineapple juice
2 tbsp apple cider vinegar
½ cup brown sugar

Directions:

1. Preheat air fryer to 360 F. In a bowl, mix in ketchup, pineapple juice, sugar, apple vinegar, and ginger. Heat the sauce in a pan over low heat.

2. Cover the chicken with the soy sauce and sherry; pour the hot sauce on top. Let sit for 15 minutes. Place the chicken in the air fryer and cook for 15 minutes. Serve.

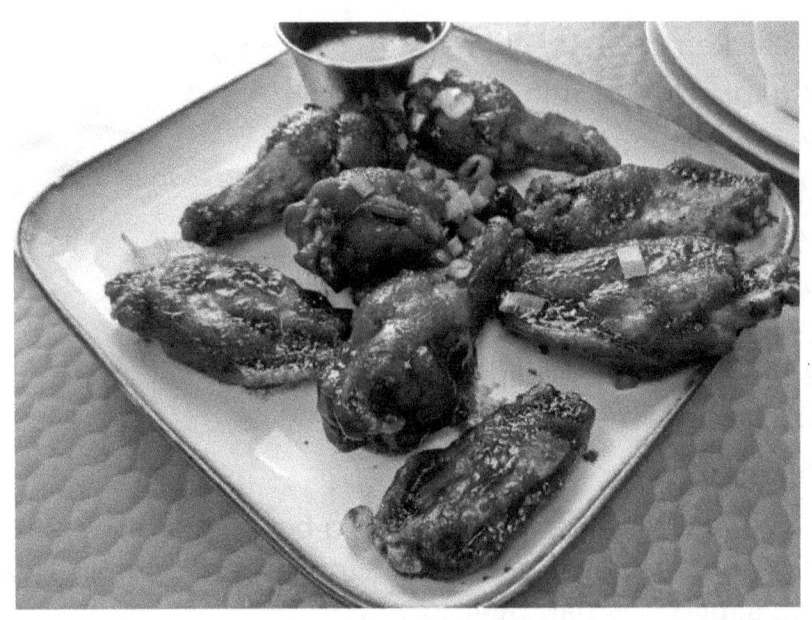

Garlicky Chicken on Green Bed

Cooking Time:

20 minutes

Serve: 4

Ingredients:

½ cup baby spinach

½ cup romaine lettuce, shredded

3 large kale leaves, chopped

1 chicken breast, cut into cubes

2 tbsp olive oil

1 tsp balsamic vinegar

1 garlic clove, minced

Salt and black pepper to taste

Directions:

1.Preheat air fryer to 390 F. In a bowl, add chicken, 1 tbsp olive oil, salt, garlic, and black pepper; mix well.

2.Pour the mixture into a baking dish and fit in the fryer. Bake for 14 minutes. In a bowl, mix the greens, remaining olive oil, and balsamic vinegar and toss to coat. Place the chicken on top and serve.

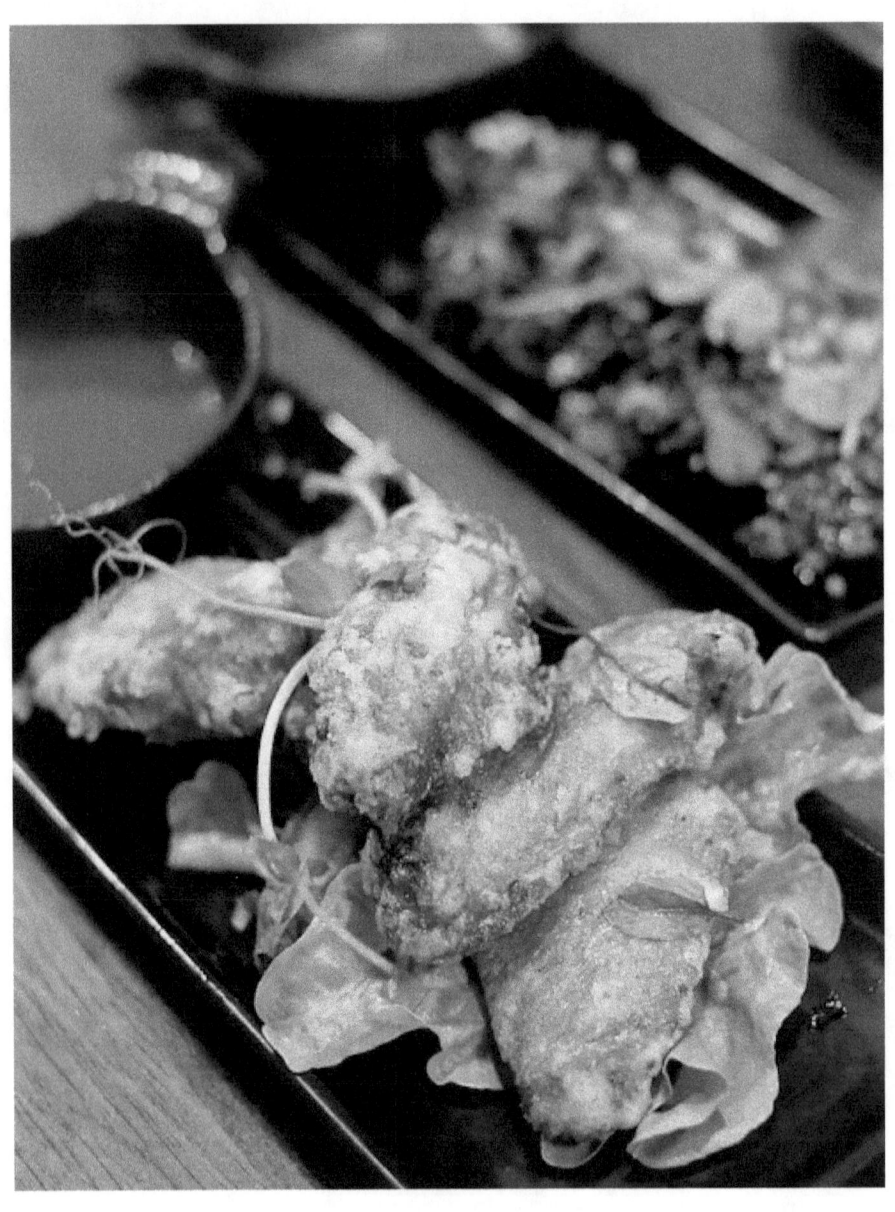

Hot Green Curry Chicken Drumsticks

Cooking Time:

20minutes

Serve:4

Ingredients:

4 chicken drumsticks, boneless, skinless
2 tbsp green curry paste
3 tbsp coconut cream
Salt and black pepper to taste
½ fresh habanero pepper, finely chopped
2 tbsp fresh parsley, roughly chopped

Directions:

1.In a bowl, mix green curry paste, coconut cream, salt, black pepper, and habanero pepper.

2.Add in the chicken drumsticks and toss to coat. Arrange the drumsticks in the greased air fryer and Bake for 13-16 minutes at 400 F, flipping once halfway through. Serve sprinkled with fresh parsley.

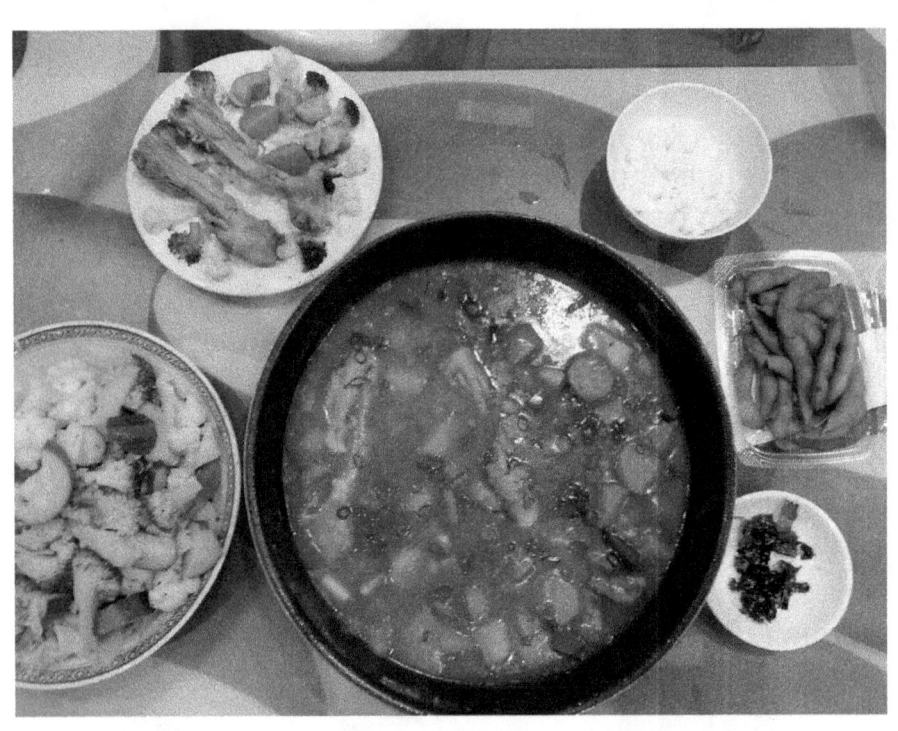

Whole Chicken with Sage & Garlic

Cooking Time:

50 minutes

Servings: 4

Ingredients:

1 3 lb whole chicken

2 tbsp olive oil

Salt and black pepper to taste

1 cup breadcrumbs

⅓ cup sage, chopped

4 cloves garlic, crushed

1 onion, chopped

3 tbsp butter

2 eggs, beaten

Directions:

1. Melt butter in a pan over medium heat and sauté garlic and onion until browned, about 5 minutes. Add in eggs, sage, black pepper, and salt; mix well.

2. Cook for 20 seconds and turn the heat off. Fill the chicken cavity with the mixture.

3. Tie the legs with a butcher's twine and brush with olive oil. Rub the top and sides of the chicken generously with salt and black pepper.

4.Preheat air fryer to 390 F. Place the chicken into the frying basket and Bake for 25 minutes.

5.Turn the chicken over and continue cooking for 10-15 more minutes, checking regularly to ensure it doesn't dry or overcooks. After, wrap in aluminum foil and let rest for 10 minutes. Carve and serve.

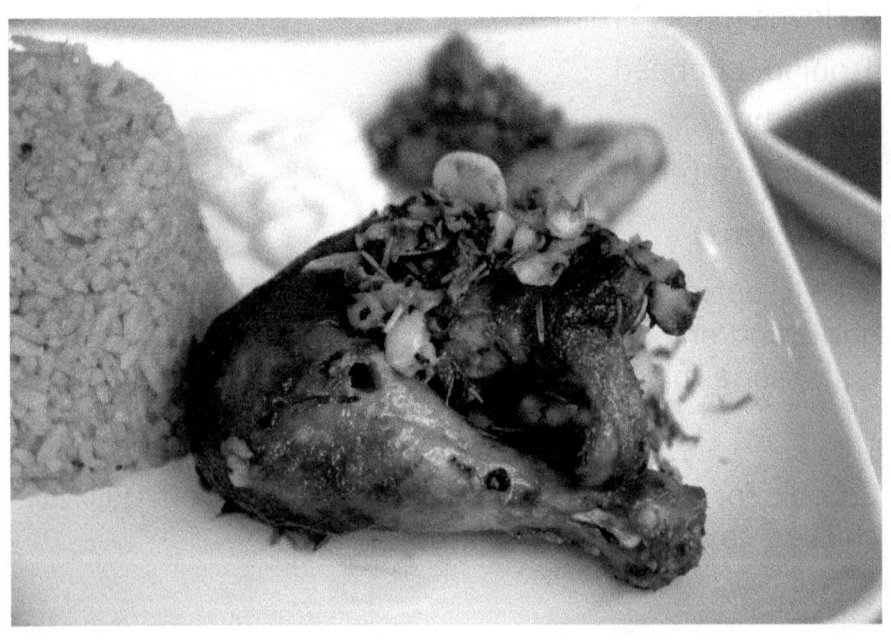

Parmesan Turkey Meatballs

Cooking Time:

25minutes

Serve:4

Ingredients:

1lb ground turkey

1 egg

½ cup breadcrumbs

1 tbsp garlic powder

1 tbsp Italian seasoning

1 tbsp onion powder

¼ cup Parmesan cheese

Salt and black pepper to taste

Directions:

1.Preheat air fryer to 400 F. In a bowl, mix ground turkey, egg, breadcrumbs, garlic powder, onion powder, Italian seasoning, Parmesan cheese, salt, and pepper. Make bite-sized balls out of the mixture.

2.Add the balls to the greased frying basket and Air Fry for 12-14 minutes, shaking once halfway through

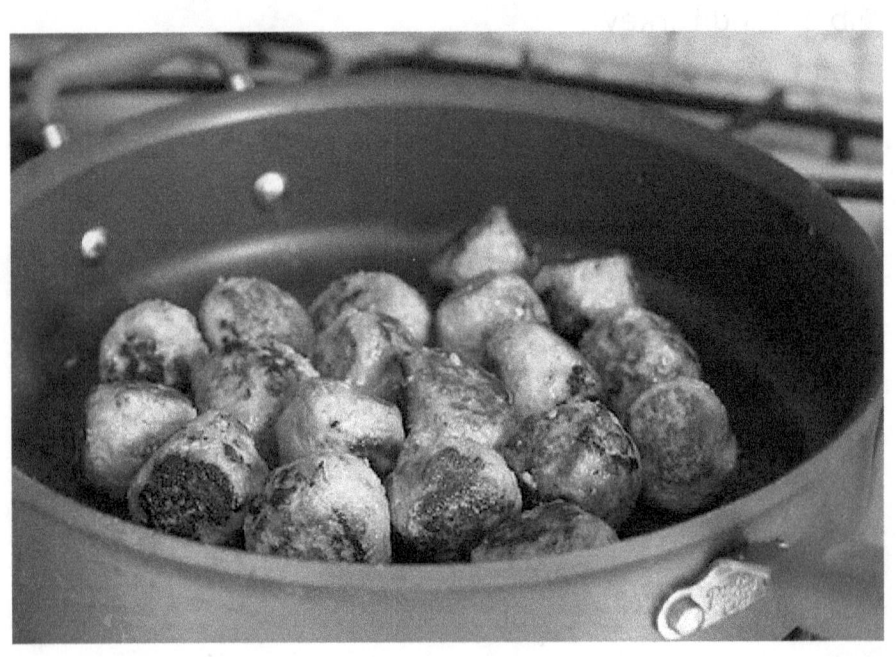

Turkey Stuffed Bell Peppers

Cooking Time:
35 minutes
Serve: 4
Ingredients:
1tbsp olive oil
½ lb ground turkey
4 bell peppers, stems and seeds removed
1 cup mozzarella cheese, shredded
1 7- oz can black beans, drained and rinsed
1 cup cooked long-grain brown rice
½ cup kernel corn
1 cup mild salsa
1 tsp chili powder
½ tsp ground cumin
2 tbsp chopped fresh cilantro
Salt and black pepper to taste

Directions:
1. Preheat air fryer to 360 F. Warm the olive oil in a large skillet over medium heat.

2. Cook the turkey, breaking it up, until browned, about 5-6 minutes. Drain any excess fat and set aside.

3. Combine the browned turkey, black beans, cheddar cheese, rice, corn, salsa, chili powder, salt, cumin, and black pepper in a bowl, then spoon the mixture into the bell peppers.

4.Put the stuffed peppers in the greased fryer basket. Bake for about 10-15 minutes. Garnish with cilantro and serve.

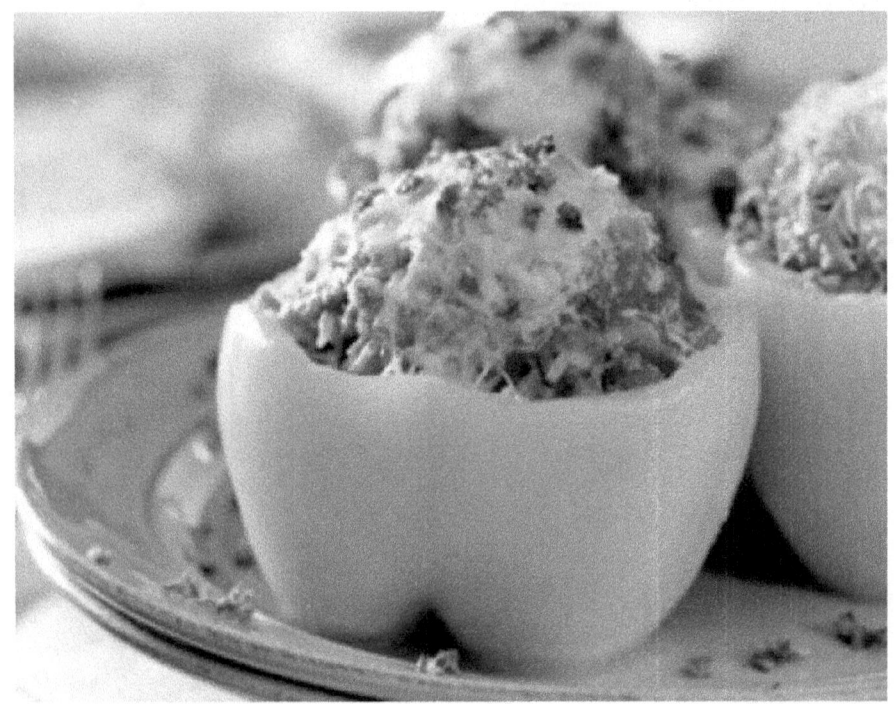

Authentic Mongolian Chicken Wings

Cooking Time:

15 minutes

Servings: 4

Ingredients:

1 lb chicken wings

1 cup flour

1 cup breadcrumbs

3 eggs, beaten

4 tbsp canola oil

Salt and black pepper to taste

2 tbsp sesame seeds

2 tbsp red pepper paste

1 tbsp apple cider vinegar

1 tbsp honey

1 tbsp soy sauce

Directions:

1. Preheat air fryer to 350 F. Separate the chicken wings into winglets and drummettes.

2. In a bowl, mix salt, olive oil, and black pepper. Coat the chicken with flour, dip in the beaten eggs, and then in the breadcrumbs.

3. Place the chicken in the frying basket and Air Fry for 15 minutes, shaking once.

4. Mix red pepper paste, vinegar, soy sauce, honey, and ¼ cup of water in a saucepan and bring to a boil. Simmer for 5-7 minutes until thickened. Pour the chicken over and sprinkle with sesame seeds. Serve.

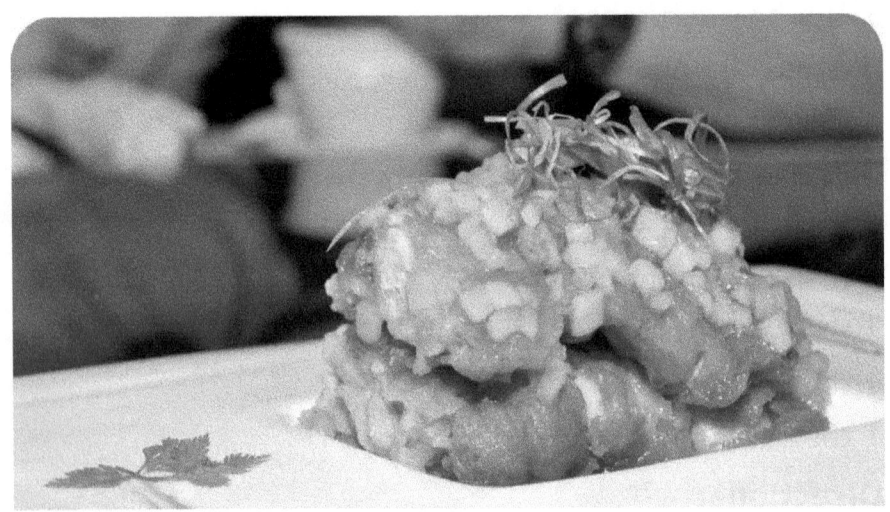

Spiced Chicken Tacos

Cooking Time:

25 minutes

Serve:6

Ingredients:

1 tbsp buffalo sauce
2 cups shredded cooked chicken
8 oz cream cheese, softened
1 tbsp olive oil
1 tsp ground cumin
½ tsp smoked paprika
12 flour tortillas

Directions:

1.Preheat air fryer to 360 F. Stir the cream cheese and Buffalo sauce in a bowl until well- combined, then add the chicken and stir some more.

2.On a clean workspace, lay the tortillas out flat and spoon 2-3 tablespoons of the chicken mixture down each tortilla center.

3.Sprinkle with cumin and smoked paprika. Roll them up and put them in the air fryer, seam side down.

4.Spray each tortilla with olive oil and air fry 5-10 minutes or until lightly golden and crisp. Arrange the tacos on plates and serve.

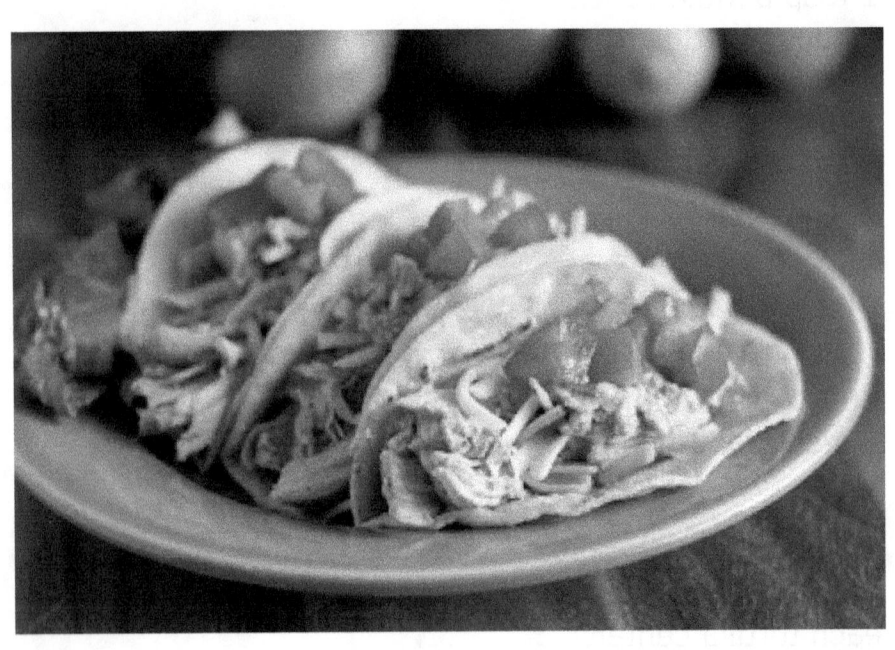

Harissa Chicken Sticks

Cooking Time:

20 minutes

Servings: 4

Ingredients:

4 chicken tenders, cut into strips

½ tsp ground cumin seeds

1 tbsp harissa powder

Salt and black pepper to taste

4 cup panko breadcrumbs

1 tbsp fresh parsley, chopped

2 large eggs, beaten

Directions:

1. Preheat air fryer to 400 F. In a bowl, mix breadcrumbs, harissa powder, cumin, salt, and black pepper.

2. Dip the chicken strips in eggs and dredge in the harissa-crumb mixture. Place in the greased frying basket and Air Fry for 15 minutes, flipping once halfway through. Serve immediately. Yummy!

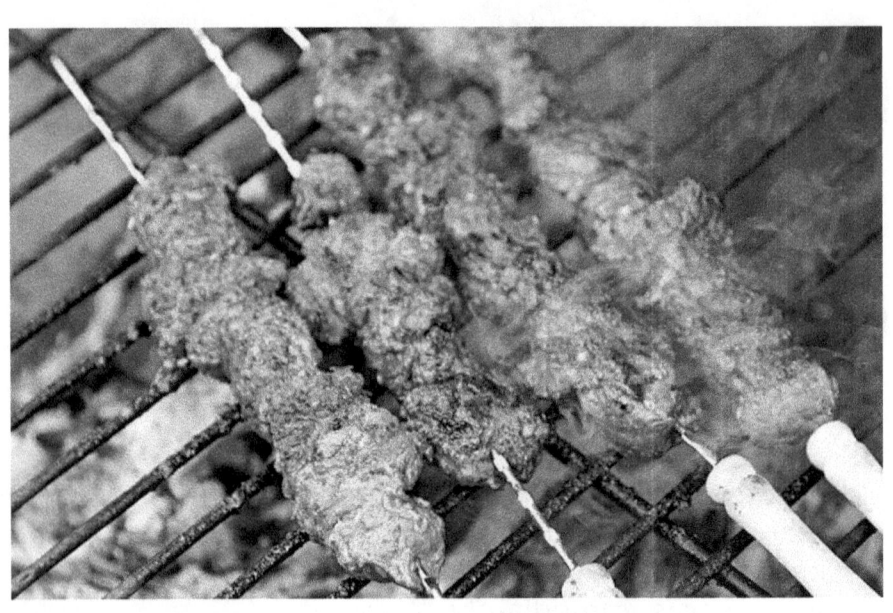

Chicken Breasts en Papillote

Cooking Time:
15 minutes
Servings: 4

Ingredients:
1 lb chicken breasts
2 tbsp butter, melted
Salt and black pepper to taste
½ tsp dried marjoram

Directions:
1. Preheat air fryer to 380 F. Place each chicken breast on a 12x12 inches aluminum foil wrap, and season with salt and black pepper.

2. Top with marjoram and butter and wrap the foil around the breasts in a loose way to create a flow of air. Bake the in the fryer for 15 minutes. Unwrap, let cool, and serve.

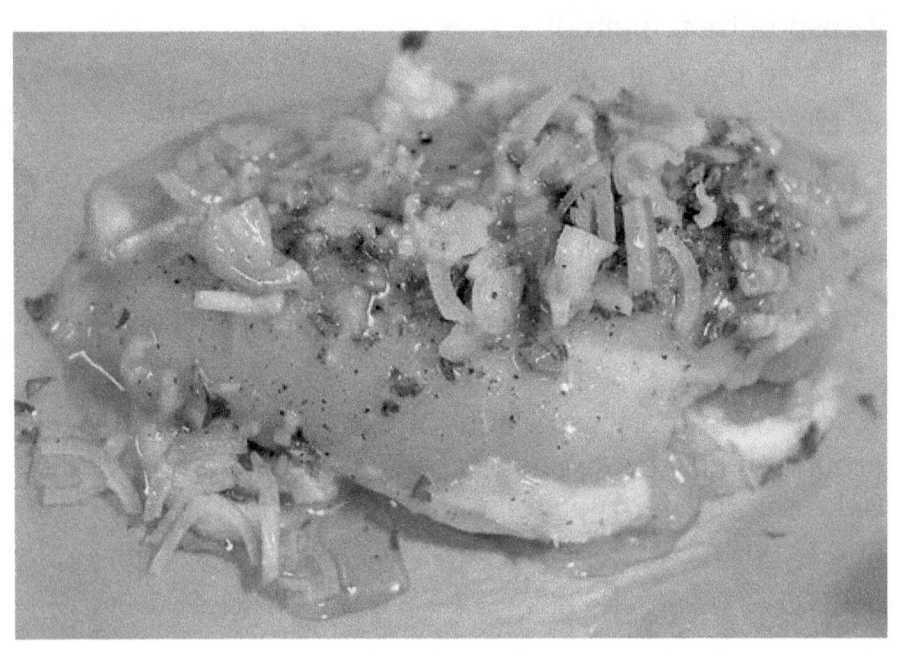

Paprika Chicken Breasts

Cooking Time:

25 minutes

Serve: 4

Ingredients:

4 chicken breasts

Salt and black pepper to taste

¼ tsp garlic powder

1 tbsp paprika

2 tbsp butter, melted

2 tbsp fresh thyme, chopped

Directions:

1. Preheat air fryer to 360 F. Grease the frying basket with cooking spray.

2. Rub the chicken with salt, black pepper, garlic powder, and paprika. Brush with butter.

3. Place in the air fryer and Air Fry for 15 minutes, flipping once halfway through cooking. Let cool slightly, then slice, and sprinkle with thyme to serve.

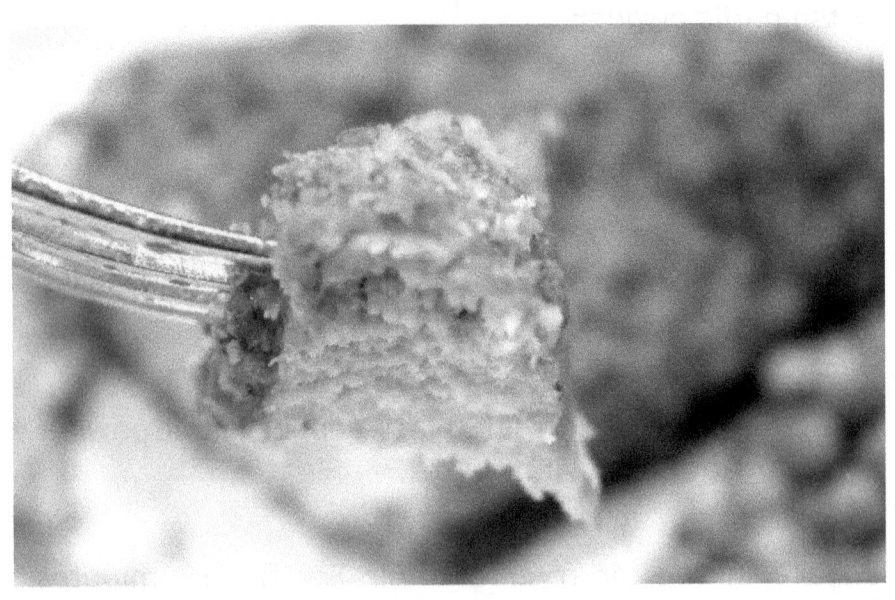

Caprese Chicken with Balsamic Sauce

Cook Time:

25 minutes

Servings:4

Ingredients:

4 chicken breasts, cubed

6 basil leaves, chopped

¼ cup balsamic vinegar

4 tomato slices

1 tbsp butter, melt

4 fresh mozzarella cheese slices

Directions:

1.Preheat the air fryer to 400 F. Mix butter and balsamic vinegar and pour it over the chicken in a bowl.

2.Let marinate for 30 minutes. Place the chicken in the frying basket and Air Fry for 14-16 minutes, shaking once. Serve topped with basil, tomato, and fresh mozzarella cheese slices

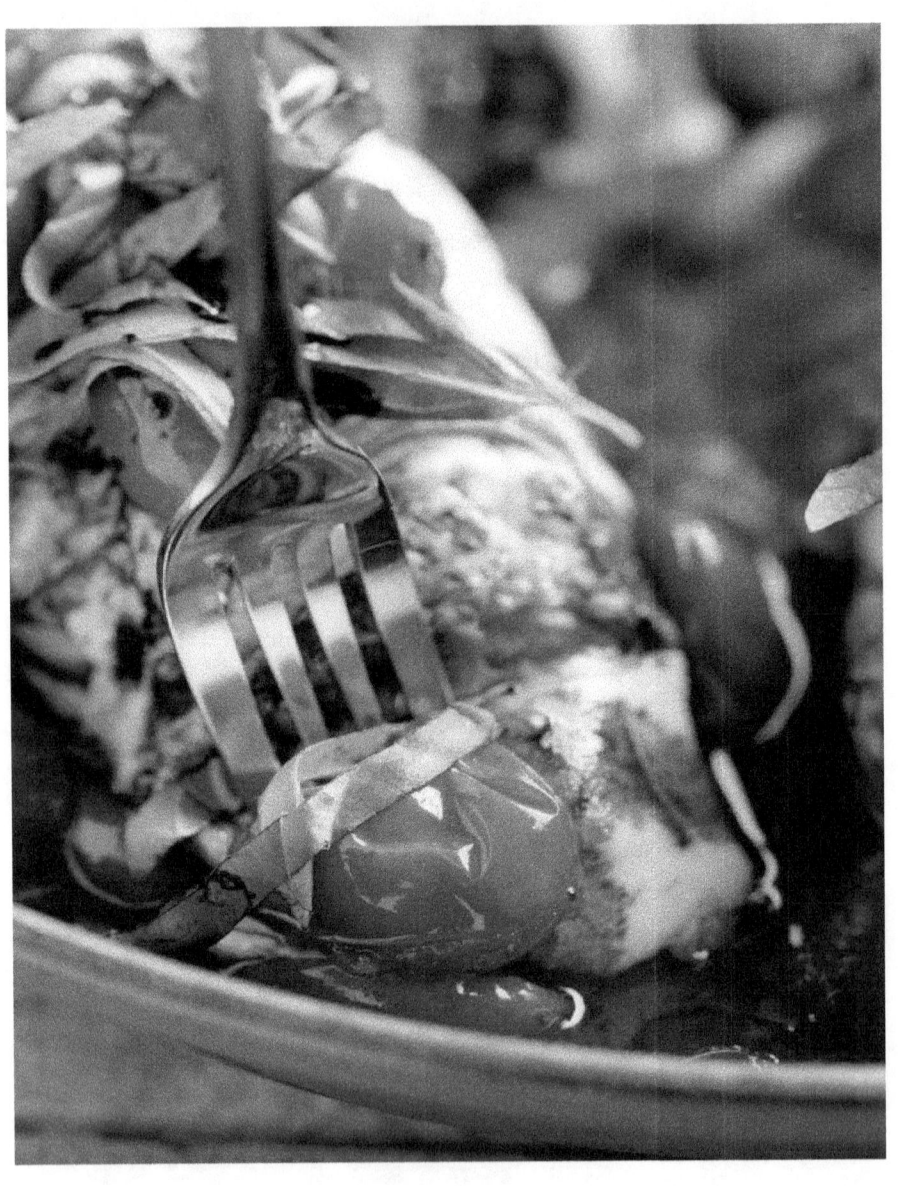

Buttermilk Chicken Thighs

Cook Time:
25 minutes
Servings: 4
INGREDIENTS

½ lb chicken thighs
½ tbsp cayenne pepper
Salt and black pepper to taste
1 cup flour
½ tsp paprika
½ tsp baking powder
2 cups buttermilk

Directions:

1. Place the chicken thighs in a bowl. Stir in cayenne, salt, pepper, and buttermilk. Refrigerate for 2 hours. Preheat air fryer to 350 F.

2. In another bowl, mix flour, paprika, salt, and baking powder.

3. Dredge the chicken thighs in the flour, and then place them on a lined baking dish.

4. Bake inside the fryer for 16-18 minutes, flipping once halfway through cooking. Serve hot.

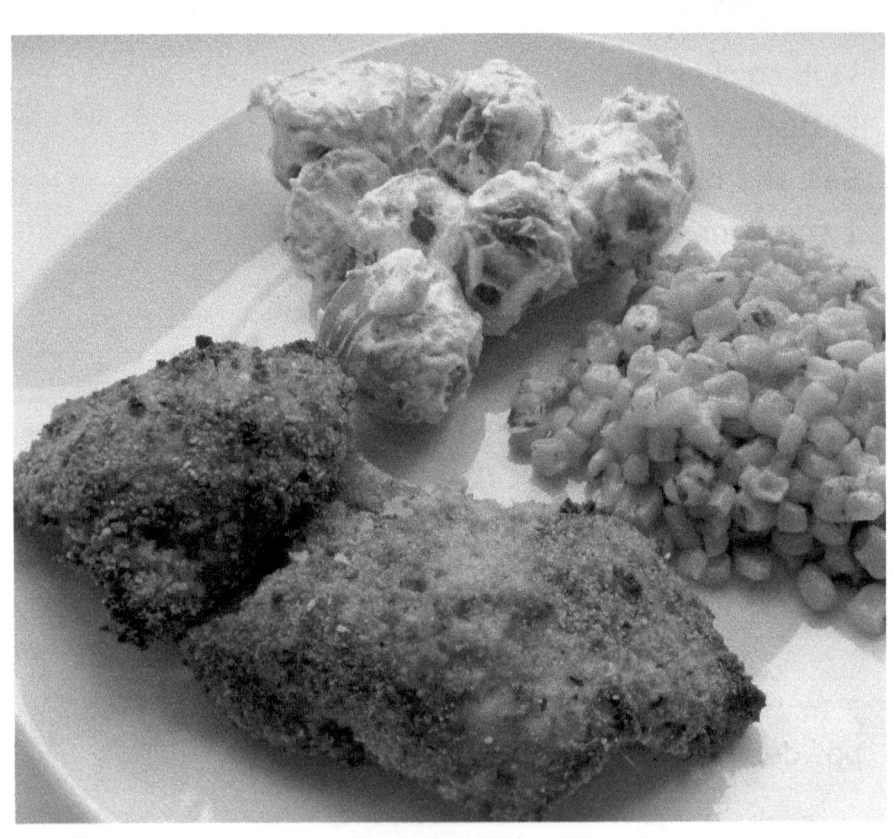

Sweet & Sticky Chicken Drumsticks

Cook Time:

20 minutes

Servings: 2

Ingredients

chicken drumsticks, skin removed
2 tbsp canola oil
1 tbsp Agave nectar
1 garlic clove, minced

Directions:

1. Add all ingredients to a resealable bag and massage until well-coated. Allow the chicken to marinate for 30 minutes.

2. Preheat the air fryer to 380 F. Add the chicken to the frying basket and Bake for 15 minutes, shaking once. Serve warm

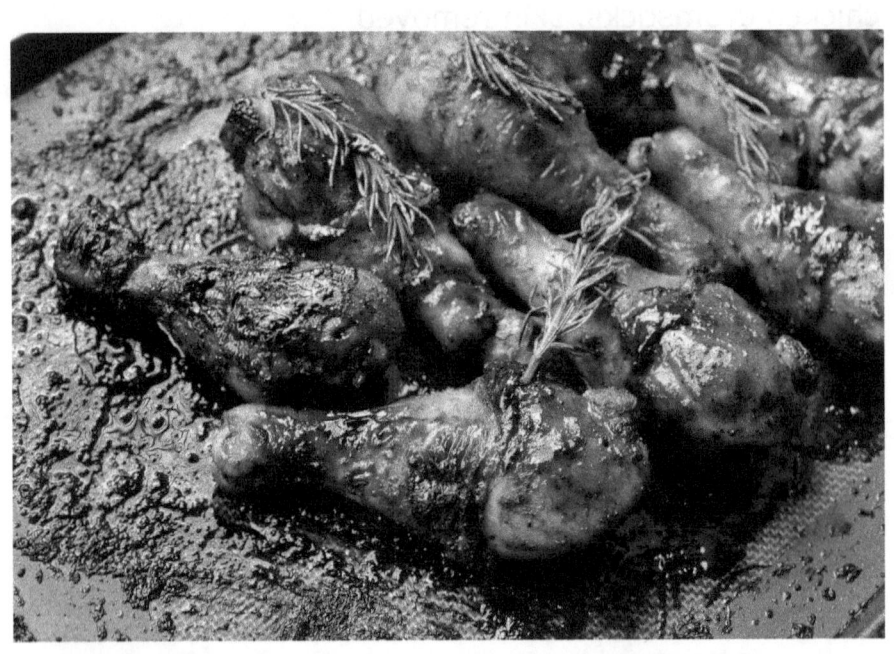

Turkey Fingers with Cranberry Glaze

Cooking Time:

20 minutes

Serve: 4

Ingredients:

1 lb turkey breast, cut into strips
1 tbsp chicken seasoning
Salt and black pepper to taste
½ cup cranberry sauce

Directions:

1. Preheat air fryer to 390 F. Season the turkey with chicken seasoning, salt, and pepper.

2. Spray with cooking spray and Air Fry in the frying basket for 10-12 minutes, flipping once halfway through.

3. Put a saucepan over low heat, and add the cranberry sauce and ¼ cup of water. Simmer for 5 minutes, stirring continuously.

4. Serve the turkey drizzled with cranberry sauce. Yummy!

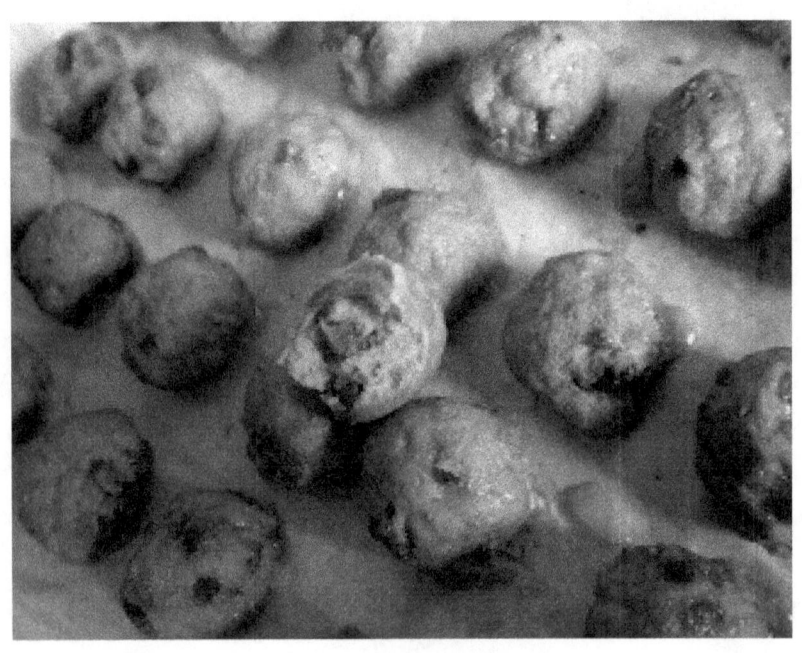

Chicken Skewers with Yogurt Dip

Cook Time:
20 minutes
Servings:4
Ingredients:

1 lb chicken tenderloins
1 tsp ground ginger
¼ cup soy sauce
1 tbsp white vinegar
1 tbsp honey
1 tbsp toasted sesame oil
2 tsp toasted sesame seeds
4 tbsp Greek yogurt
2 tbsp fresh cilantro, chopped
1 lime, zested and juiced
2 tbsp sweet chili sauce
8 wooden skewer, soaked in water for 30 minutes

Directions:

1. Combine the soy sauce, white vinegar, honey, sesame oil, lime juice, and ginger in a zip-top bag to make a marinade.

2. Toss the chicken in the bag, seal it, and put it in the fridge for a minimum of 2 hours to as long as overnight to marinate.

3. Combine the Greek yogurt, cilantro, lime zest, and the remaining lime juice in a small bowl and mix to combine.

4. Keep in the fridge until ready to use. Preheat air fryer to 380 F. Skewer each tenderloin on the wooden skewer and sprinkle with sesame seeds.

5. Keep the excess marinade. Put the skewers in a single layer in the greased fryer basket and air fry for 6 minutes, flip the chicken, baste with more marinade, and cook 5-8 more minutes or until crispy.

6. Serve the skewers hot with the yogurt dip on the side.

Popcorn Chicken Tenders

Cooking Time:

20 minutes

Servings: 4

Ingredients:

1lb chicken tenders, cut into strips
½ cup cooked popcorn
½ cup panko breadcrumbs
2 eggs
4 tbsp corn flour
½ tsp dried oregano
2 tbsp butter, melted
Salt and black pepper to taste

Directions:

1. Preheat the air fryer to 400 F. Pulse the popcorn in a blender until crumbs-like texture.

2. In a bowl, combine the corn flour, oregano, salt, and black pepper. In another bowl, beat the eggs with some salt. In a third, mix panko crumbs with popcorn crumbs.

3. Dip the chicken strips in the flour, then in the egg, and then coat with the breadcrumbs. Place in the air fryer basket.

4. Drizzle with the melted butter and Air Fry for 12-14 minutes, flipping once halfway through. Serve.

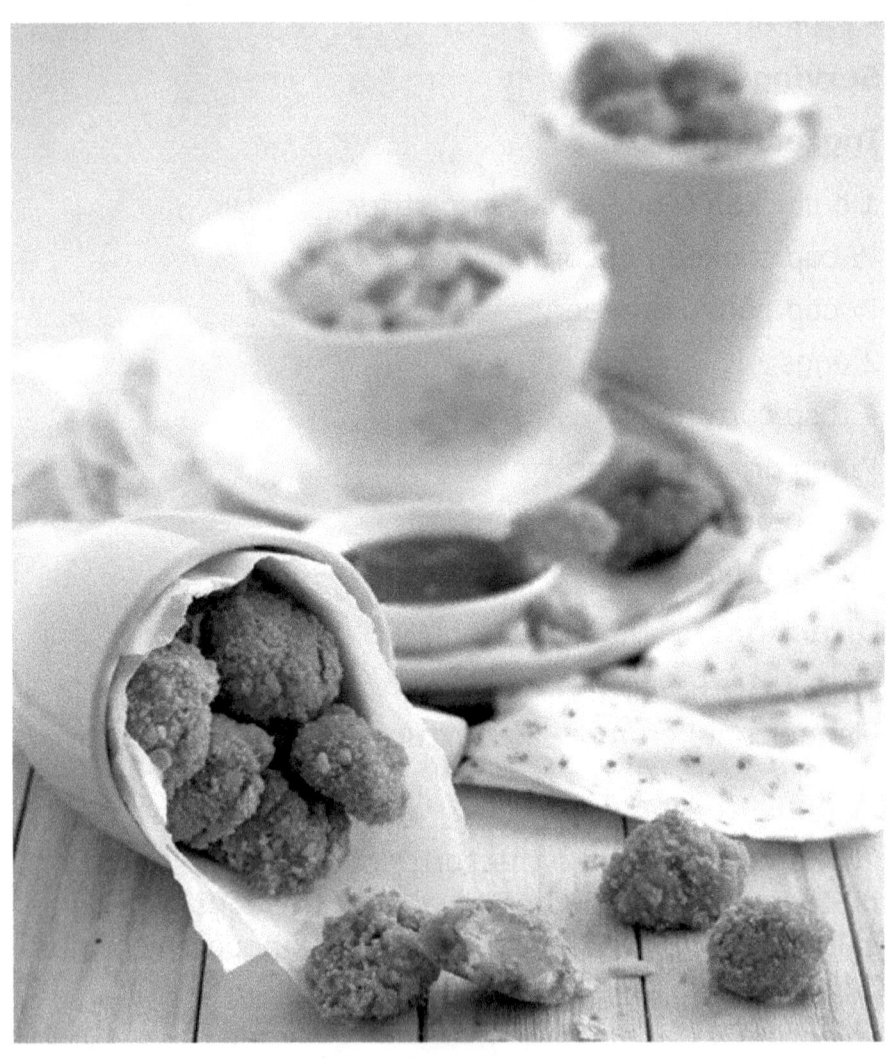

www.ingramcontent.com/pod-product-compliance
Lightning Source LLC
Chambersburg PA
CBHW071109030426
42336CB00013BA/2015